KU-213-990

before

This

LOST CIRCULATION

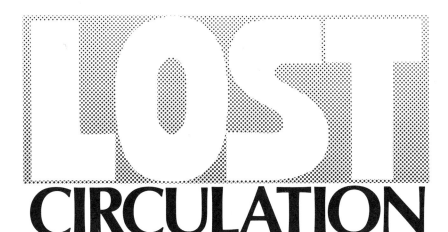

CIRCULATION

Joseph U. Messenger

PennWell Books
PennWell Publishing Company
Tulsa, Oklahoma

05764191

Copyright © 1981 by
PennWell Publishing Company
1421 South Sheridan Road/P.O. Box 1260
Tulsa, Oklahoma 74101

Library of Congress Cataloging in Publication Data
Messenger, Joseph U.
   Lost circulation.
   Bibliography: p. 108
   Includes index.
   1. Oil well drilling—Lost circulation.
I. Title.
TN871.2.M377   622'.338   81-11950
ISBN 0-87814-175-8   AACR2

D
622.3382
MES

Printed in the United States of America

1 2 3 4 5   85 84 83 82 81

iv

Table of Contents

INTRODUCTION

Lost circulation is the most troublesome and costly problem in drilling for oil. Yearly costs in materials, lost rig time, and lost holes amount to millions of dollars.* Yet no functionally new lost circulation materials or techniques have been developed in the past ten years. However, progress has been made by using existing materials and techniques more effectively. Emphasis has been placed on using cheap materials that are commonly stocked at rigs and therefore easily available.

In this book, the types of loss zones are described and classified on the basis of severity, and the different materials and techniques are detailed and matched functionally to the type and severity of the zone they most likely can cure. The mechanisms by which loss zones are sealed are described. A list of the most usual causes of failure to cure losses is presented. In addition, attention is given to methods of preventing lost circulation. It has been estimated that 50% of all lost circulation could be prevented by good drilling and good drilling mud practices.†

Indefensibly absent from prior treatments of lost circulation are materials and techniques where oil muds are used. In all cases in this book, the materials and techniques are evaluated as to whether they have direct application in oil muds. And barite plugs and barite-in-oil plugs are described, as is their application for controlling wells that are kicking while loss zones are sealed.

---

*J. L. Lummus, "New Material Proves Successful to Stop Lost Circulation under Various Conditions," *Petroleo Interamericano*, December 1966, p. 26; Magcobar, "Free-World Sale of Lost-Circulation Materials."
†B.Q. Green, "Eight Steps to Stop Lost Circulation," *Pet Eng.*, March 1963, p. 74.

CHAPTER 1
What is Lost Circulation?

Lost circulation, or lost returns, is the loss to formation voids of whole drilling fluid or cement slurry used during drilling operations. The loss may vary from a gradual lowering of the pits to a complete loss of returns. (Reductions in mud volume due to loss of filtrate from the mud or filling new hole should not be confused with lost circulation.)

Mud losses vary in type, severity, and location in the hole. Even with experience in an area, it is difficult to make valid blanket recommendations. But there is a systematic approach to controlling lost circulation that uses the most economic and effective method known immediately. This approach involves both preventive and corrective measures. It is particularly concerned with the correct use of lost circulation materials such as bentonite, diesel oil and cement and a blend of bridging agents that must be stocked on every location.

Types of Loss Zones

Mud losses can occur to six types of formations: 1) unconsolidated or highly permeable formations (loose gravels), 2) natural fractures, 3) horizontal induced fractures, 4) cavernous formations (crevices and channels), and 5) vertical natural and induced fractures.[1] Broadly, loss zones are either horizontal or vertical. Induced and natural fractures are horizontal to depths of 2,500–4,000 feet; below this depth, they are vertical. To induce horizontal fractures, the rock strength and the overburden pressure must be overcome. This requires a mud weight equivalent of 19.4 lb/gal or greater. Since vertical fractures occur without lifting the overburden, they can be induced at much lower pressures.

The following loss zones are listed in order of increasing severity. The identifying features of each are shown in Tables 1–1 and 1–2.

Horizontal Loss Zones

Porous sands and gravels (Fig. 1–1). In order for the matrix of a porous formation to accept whole mud or cement, it must have a permeability of 10–100 darcies. Shallow sands and gravels often have such permeabilities and therefore can accept whole mud or cement. However, deep sands usually do not have permeabilities over 3.5 darcies.

TABLE 1–1 Identifying Features of Horizontal Loss Zones (After Howard and Scott, Messenger)

Porous Sands and Gravels	Natural Fractures	Induced Fractures	Cavernous Zones
1. Gradual lowering of mud level in pits.	1. May occur in any type rock.	1. Occur where fractures are horizontal in any formation under mud rings.	1. Normally confined to limestone.
2. Losses may become complete if drilling is continued.	2. Loss is evidenced by gradual lowering of the mud in the pits. If drilling is continued and more fractures are exposed, complete loss of returns may be experienced.	2. Marked increase in pump pressure.	2. Loss of returns may be sudden and complete.
3. Since rock permeability must exceed about 10 darcies before whole mud can penetrate and oil and gas sand permeability seldom exceeds about 3.5 darcies, it is improbable that loose sands are the cause of mud loss to an oil or gas sand unless the loss can be attributed to the ease with which this type of formation fractures.	3. Fracture must have a finite supported width to take mud.	3. Drillstring becomes tight.	3. Bit may drop several inches to several feet just preceding loss.
		4. Can occur in poorly compacted sea-bed formations in offshore drilling because of a gradual mud weight buildup.	4. Drilling may be rough before loss.

TABLE 1-2   Identifying Features of Vertical Loss Zones

Natural Fractures	Induced Fractures	Underground Blowout
1. May occur in any type rock. 2. Loss will go from partial to complete as more formation is drilled, particularly if drilling is accompanied by an increase in mud weight.	1. May occur in any type rock but would be expected below 2,500 feet. 2. Loss is usually sudden and accompanied by complete loss of returns. Conditions are conducive to forming induced fractures when mud weight exceeds 10.5 ppg. 3. Loss may follow any sudden surge of pressure or trip. 4. When loss of circulation occurs and adjacent wells have not experienced lost circulation, induced fractures should be expected.	1. Condition where fluids flow from a lower active zone to an upper induced vertical fracture. 2. Evidenced by unstable pressure readings and by an inexplicable change in pressures and mud volumes. 3. Should be expected if good kill operations fail to control the well.

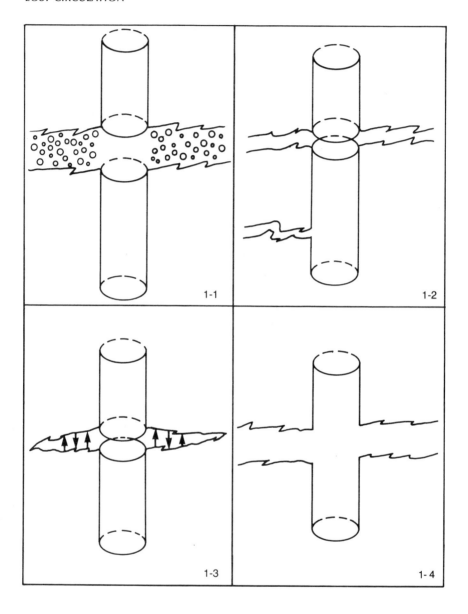

Fig. 1–1   Horizontal loss zone: porous sands and gravels
Fig. 1–2   Horizontal loss zone: natural or intrinsic fracture
Fig. 1–3   Induced horizontal fracture
Fig. 1–4   Cavernous formations

Hence, their matricies are rarely loss zones unless they are fractured. Porous gravels lie horizontally and support the overburden. The pores of the gravel, not the widening, constitute the loss zone. They can be filled with air or water of varying pressures. To widen a gravel, its overburden must be lifted. This is not likely to occur at shallow depths.

Natural or intrinsic horizontal fractures (Fig. 1–2). For a natural horizontal fracture to exist, the overburden must be self-supporting. This is true whether the fracture is ¼ inch wide or 100 feet wide. To widen a natural horizontal fracture, the overburden must be lifted. The fracture can be filled with water or air so the hole can empty the drilling mud into it.

Induced horizontal fractures (Fig. 1–3). There are two to three circumstances where a horizontal fracture can be induced. The most common is in a shale (or other formation) under a mud ring. (Note: this can always be cured by removing the mud ring and allowing the overburden to subside and close the fracture.) Another type is offshore in an undercompacted sea bed. Still another is fractures that occur when drilling from a mountain top.

Cavernous formations (Fig. 1–4). A cavern is a natural fracture of very large proportions that mostly occurs in limestones. Cavernous formations are horizontal and the overburden is self-supporting. Water can be flowing in horizontal fractures or caverns both within the fracture or from an upper or lower zone into them, making them more difficult to seal.

Vertical Loss Zones

Natural vertical fractures (Fig. 1–5). Natural vertical fractures do exist in formations below 2,500 feet. However, while the fracture is there, it has little or no width. Therefore, mud losses to them are slight until they are widened into induced fractures. This is more easily accomplished than for horizontally induced fractures. Since the fracture already exists, only the fracture propagation pressure must be overcome to open and extend it.

Induced vertical fractures (Fig. 1–6). While mud losses to caverns are the most difficult to overcome, they are not the most prevalent. Caverns occur mostly in limestones, but mud losses to induced vertical fractures can occur in essentially any formation—a troublesome situation. Conditions that may help induce fractures are well irregularities, high mud weight, excessive back pressure or chokedown, rough handling of the drilling tools, and a closed hydraulic system.

Underground blowout (Fig. 1–7). An underground blowout is a condition where fluids (usually gas or water) are flowing from a lower

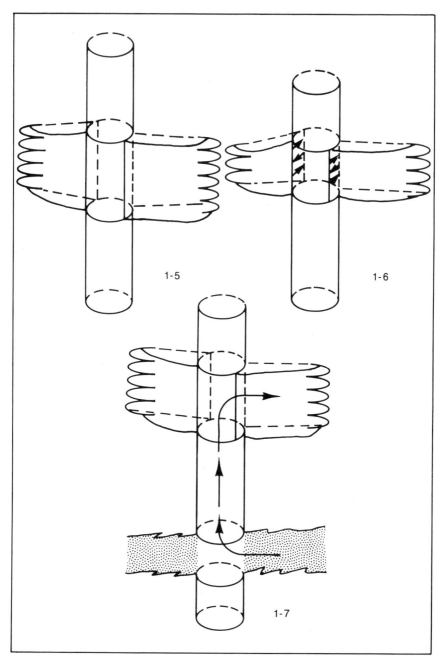

1-5

1-6

1-7

Fig. 1–5 Natural vertical fractures
Fig. 1–6 Induced vertical fractures

Fig. 1–7 Underground blowout

active zone into a higher loss zone (usually an induced vertical fracture).

Induced vertical fractures differ from natural vertical fractures in that loss of mud to induced vertical fractures requires enough pressure to break or split the formation. The loss of mud to natural vertical fractures requires only sufficient pressure to exceed the fracture propagation pressure.

Natural fractures can be widened by excessive overpressure; they then behave as induced vertical fractures. It is more difficult to prevent mud losses to induced vertical fractures because pressures exceeding those at which they were sealed will widen the fracture and thereby destroy the seal.

Induced vertical fractures are the most troublesome because they can occur in essentially every type of formation below 2,500 feet. To induce a vertical fracture, the rock strength and the fracture propagation pressure must be exceeded. Thereafter, the fracture propagation pressure is all that is required to widen and extend the fracture. As long as its fracture propagation pressure is exceeded, an induced vertical fracture is limitless.

CHAPTER 2
Lost Circulation Prevention

The two most common but avoidable causes of lost circulation are excessive downhole pressures and setting intermediate (protective) casing too high.

Controlling Downhole Pressures

Excessive downhole pressures can arise from several sources. Of these, perhaps the most important is the hydrostatic pressure produced by the column of mud. The hydrostatic head of a column of mud necessary to offset formation-fluid pressures may fracture upper formations. This can result in a dangerous kick with simultaneous loss of returns.

Another source of pressure is the mud circulating density. This is the pressure required to overcome the inertia of the mud column and the friction of the mud against the sides of the hole. Other factors adding to circulation density are a high circulation rate, surging the pumps, and rough, quick handling of the drillstring. Still another source is restrictions in the annulus from swollen casing protectors, mud-cake buildup, excessive cuttings from drilling too fast, cuttings collecting in hole enlargements, and balled-up drill tools.

These contributors to downhole pressure problems can be minimized by observing the following precautionary measures:

1. Minimize hydrostatic pressure. The hydrostatic pressure of the mud column can be minimized by drilling with the lowest safe mud weight. Particularly in wildcat wells, drilling underbalanced should be avoided because kicks put uncontrollably high pressures on the open formations and cause lost returns. In areas where lost circulation can occur, drilling should be balanced using the minimum safe mud weight.

2. Minimize circulating density. Lowering the mud weight lowers inertia. The friction of the mud against the sides of the hole can be lowered by adjusting the mud properties (viscosity, yield point, and gel strength) within safe limits. If the yield point of the mud is sufficient, high circulation rates will not be required to clean the hole.

The pump surges and rough, quick handling of the drillstring are completely controllable by the drill crew. They are easily avoided by:

a) taking 45–60 seconds to raise or lower a stand
b) drilling, not spudding, all bridges

c) breaking circulation cautiously after engaging the rotary and while slowly pulling up the drillpipe (Note: do not speed up the pump until circulation has been established and the bit is on bottom)

d) slowing the mud pumps as much as is practical

A driller warning system is recommended for preventing unnecessary downhole pressure surges. A light or horn warns the driller if he moves the string too fast. Several types are presently available on the market.

Avoid plugging the bit, perhaps by always running a float. The common method for unplugging bits may still be spudding the drillstring. The pressure surges from it are bound to break down the open formations.

3. Avoid restrictions in the annulus. One of the ways to avoid hangups is to drill a straight, clean, stabilized hole of adequate size at the optimum rate. But what if a crooked, dirty, washed-out, unstable hole is unavoidable? In this case, stabilized hole can also be drilled. Start with a circulation rate that is adequate to clean the hole and drill it of an adequate size at a controlled rate. Dirty or not, the hole will gradually stabilize. Once it has, stability is maintained keeping that rate of circulation whatever the operation. For example, if 9⅝-inch casing is to be run in 12¼-inch hole and the hole is stabilized at a circulation rate of 120 ft/min, then the casing should be run so that this stabilized annular velocity is maintained. Also, when the cement slurry is displaced, the same 120 ft/min annular velocity should be kept. For 9⅝-inch casing in a 12¼-inch hole, this is about one-half the circulation rate used while drilling. The running rate for this should be such that the flow past the casing is the stabilized 120 ft/min. This adjustment should be made for all full-hole tools that may need to be run.

Drilling too fast causes 9 out of 10 drilling problems. A typical too-fast drilling curve is shown on page 10 in Fig. 2–1. One function of management is to define and then to take the optimum risk. Management encourages the curve from point A to point B but then goes deaf, dumb and blind when the drilling curve goes from B to C. Troubleshooters see only the BC curve, and are generally powerless to prevent it. So why don't all concerned take the optimum risk and drill at the optimum controlled rate shown by curve AEF?

The maximum cuttings a mud in ideal shape can carry is 5 vol%. Concentrations higher than this result in mud rings that ball the bit, collars, and stabilizers. Under a mud ring at any depth, circulation can be lost to an induced horizontal or vertical fracture. If the fracture is horizontal, circulation can be regained by removing the mud ring. If the fracture is vertical, particularly where an oil mud is being used, the

9

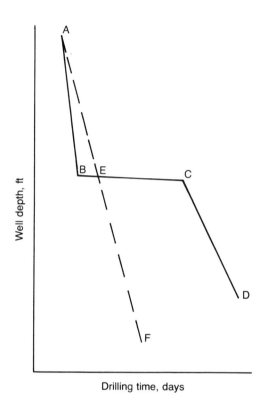

Fig. 2–1 Typical too-fast drilling curve

damage is irreversible; the fracture will not heal. In the worst cases, the fracture propagation pressure is as much as 3.0 lb/gal below the fracture initiation pressure. In other words, the damage done will have to be repaired. Below mud rings, mud can also be fraced into formations without noticeable loss of returns. Fracing mud into formations thus makes them slough and should be avoided.

In some drilling, dirty hole cannot be avoided. But by drilling and circulating at a controlled rate, the hole can be stabilized. As long as the stabilized circulation and drilling rate are maintained, the cuttings will stay put.

Mud cake buildup on porous zones can be controlled by lowering the filter loss of the mud in use. This may or may not be adequate. However, with improved mud solids-handling equipment, the particles in the drilling mud can be sized so they form an in-formation filter cake, thereby preventing much of the cake buildup on the face of the hole. Modern mud solids-handling equipment helps prevent loss of circulation and for this function alone is worth its trouble and cost.

Finally, using casing protectors that don't swell, removing those that have before they become a problem, and avoiding the use of over-sized stabilizers are straightforward means of avoiding restrictions in the annulus.

4. Other precautions. If lost-circulation zones are expected against which bridging agents are known to be effective, pretreat the mud with these materials before penetrating the loss zone. For example, if small natural fractures are expected, a bridging agent such as fine black walnut hulls will pass the shaker screen and increase the pressure required to open the fractures.

Keep adequate records. Actually, adequate records of the prevention and cure of lost circulation are rarely kept. Usually, both good and bad experience gained in an operations area leaves with the drilling personnel when they are transferred. Adequate records that describe the lost-circulation problems and the materials and techniques used to combat them are valuable—almost a necessity. A table such as the lost-circulation problem report form in Table 2–1 should be adopted by the operator and used religiously.

Setting Intermediate (Protective) Casing into Transition Zones

In most instances, mud losses in vertical induced fractures (the most troublesome and costly type of loss) occur because the protective casing was set too high and exposed a low-pressure formation that fractured when mud density was increased to control deeper, high-pressure zones. The interval where there is a gradual change from this low-pressure zone to the high-pressure one is called the *transition zone*. If the protective casing can be set into the transition zone, many of the mud losses to vertical induced fractures can be prevented.

Only recently has the significance of the transition zone been fully realized. Effective means of identifying it precisely are being developed by operating people. These involve indirect and direct means:

TABLE 2–1 Lost Circulation Report Form

DESCRIPTION OF WELL

Operator _____ Lease/Well No. _____
Fld/Town _____ Sec./T'ship/Reg. _____ County _____
State _____ Co. Rep. _____
Contractor _____ Rig. No. _____ Toolpusher _____

DESCRIPTION OF LOSS ZONE

Depth, ft. _____ Type _____ Formation _____
Severity: Am't Of Loss. bpm _____ Static Fluid Level, ft. _____
Total Mud Lost, bbl _____ Survey Used to Locate Loss _____
Operation When Loss Occurred _____
Circ. Rate bpm _____ Pump Pressure, psi _____

Job a _____ Success _____ Failure _____

Lost Circulation Remedial Techniques

Technique No.	Description	Loss Zone Type Where Technique is Effective
1.	Pull Up and Wait	Seeping, Partial, and Complete Losses to Induced Fractures
2.	Bridging Agents in Mud (Water or Oil Base)	Seeping, Partial, and Less Severe Complete Losses to both Horizontal and Vertical Loss Zones
3.	High Filter Loss Slurry Squeeze (See also Techniques 3A, 3B, and 3C)	Seeping, Partial, and Complete Losses to both Horizontal and Vertical Loss Zones
4.	Cements (Neat, 4; Extended, 4A; Thixotropic, 4B; Mix Your Own, 4C)	Complete Losses and Severe Complete Losses to Horizontal and Some Vertical Loss Zones
5.	Downhole-Mixed Soft/Hard Plugs (M-DOB2C)	Complete Losses and Severe Complete Losses to Horizontal and Vertical Loss Zones.
6.	Surface-Mixed Soft Plug (PAL-MIX 11OR)	Complete Losses to Induced Vertical Fractures. Has application in both water and oil muds
7.	Downhole-Mixed Soft Plugs (7, DOB; 7A, Bengum; 7B, Polymer Plug; 7C, OM-WOB; 7D, Flo-Chek)	Complete Losses to Induced Vertical Fractures and to hold cement slurries at or near the well bore against all complete losses. Flo-Chek has application in oil muds
8.	Specialized Agents—Water, Gelled Water, Gelled Oil Carrying Sand or Limestone	Severe Complete losses to Induced Vertical Fractures and to Losses to Productive Zones
9.	Drill Blind or with Aerated Mud and Set Pipe	Very Severe Losses to Caverns, Large Natural Horizontal Fractures, and Long Sections of Honeycomb

To develop a more complete form, see Messenger, *OGJ*, 13 May 1968, p. 76.

Indirect

From the surface using seismic data. If overpressured zones can be identified from the surface before spudding the well, drilling mud properties can be more realistically predicted and no interruption of drilling is required.

Downhole by logging data. Formation resistivity, conductivity, and density can be estimated using sonic and electric logs. Resistivity and shale density decrease in pressured zones while conductivity increases. These parameters are very reliable in picking the transition zone; however, drilling must be interrupted for them to be run.

Back-pressuring tools. Kicking wells can be shut in and flowed and the pressures measured with complete control.

Direct

Drilling parameters. The drilling parameters that identify an over-pressured (transition) zone are 1) increased drilling rate, 2) unusual hole conditions such as tight hole, sloughing, increased cuttings size, and increased volume of cuttings, and 3) mud cutting as evidenced by connection gas or kicks of gas or water.

Shale densities. The density of shale decreases from 2.4 to 2.2 SG as a pressured zone is penetrated. This decrease of shale density can be monitored at the surface using proven analytical techniques.

Differential flowline temperature. There is a marked increase in formation temperature as a pressured zone is penetrated. This is reflected while drilling it by a marked increase in flowline temperature. For the most definitive results, the differential flowline temperature (°F per 100 feet) rather than the flowline temperature in °F should be plotted against depth.

CHAPTER 3
Plugging Mechanisms

Loss zones can be separated broadly into horizontal and vertical areas. Before discussing plugging mechanisms, however, a review of the borehole geometry where a horizontal and vertical loss zone contact the well bore would be helpful.

Referring to Figs. 3–1 and 3–2, it can be seen that horizontal zones contact on a circle. The zone would be limited in height and lost circulation materials would pancake out in a horizontal plane or on the face of the hole. On the other hand, vertical loss zones contact the hole in a line and can have vertical contacts up to 500 feet in height. Lost circulation materials would flow into a vertical plane and would not pancake but would tend to drop or settle—extending rather than sealing the fracture.

Plugging Horizontal Zones
Porous Sands and Gravels

Bridging agents are effective in plugging porous sands and gravels (Fig. 3–3). Being coarser than the particles in the drilling mud, they

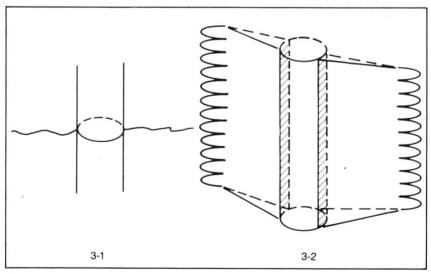

3-1   3-2

Fig. 3–1   **Horizontal contact**
Fig. 3–2   **Vertical contact**

14

collect in the interstices of the gravel, block the flow, and finally form a cake on the face of the gravel. For the seal to be permanent (that is, not to be scraped off by the bit or removed by pressure surges from the formation to the hole because the hole is swabbed or not kept full while tripping), it is best to have the cake reach into the gravel to some extent. The fiber component aids in this by binding the granular and flake bridging agents and the gravel. The examination of a gravel plugged with sawdust and shredded leather fiber showed that the leather fibers had actually done this.

Natural Horizontal Fractures

Bridging agents are effective against mud losses to natural fractures up to ¼ inch wide. However, the blend must contain a granular agent approximately the width of the fracture in size. For the fracture to be sealed, the granular agent must form a bridge at the face of or preferably out in the fracture (Fig. 3–4). The seal is more permanent if the bridge is out in the fracture and the fracture is packed with lost circulation material and mud solids by dehydration or loss of whole mud. There is little danger that the fracture can be widened since the overburden must be lifted to accomplish this. Failure usually occurs because a seal at the face is scraped off or a breakthrough of the seal in the formation occurs.

Natural horizontal fractures from ¼ inch to 1 foot in width can be sealed using cement slurries, provided the cement slurry can be held around the well bore in contact with the bottom and top of the fracture until the cement sets. To accomplish this, sometimes soft plugs are run ahead of the cement slurry to act as backup and to hold the cement slurry in place. Ideally, the cement slurry would form a perfect concentric ring around the well bore. The fact is, however, that the plug will more nearly resemble the shape shown in Fig. 3–5. Notice that on most of the circumference of the seal, the plug has little breadth. This makes it easy to destroy the plug by breaking or sucking drilling mud or formation fluids through it.

If fluids (usually water) are flowing within the fracture or from an upper zone into the fracture, the cement slurry will be washed away and no seal will be obtained. The former is indicated if circulation is restored and cement is found in the hole above the fracture. When the plug is drilled out and the fracture is reached, complete loss of circulation recurs. The latter is indicated if no cement slurry is found in the hole at all and circulation was never established.

Soft/hard and soft plugs are effective against natural horizontal fractures from ¼ inch to 1 foot wide. Because they develop high gel strength, they have more resistance to flow as they are placed and

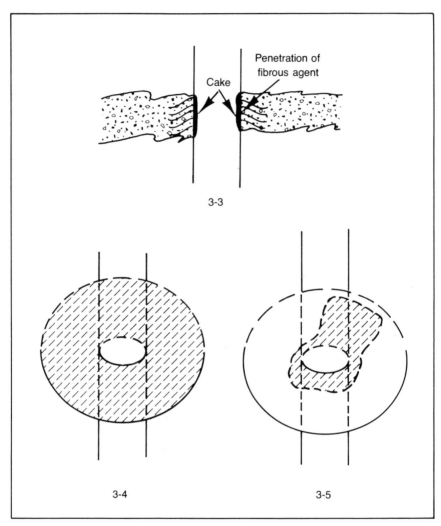

Fig. 3–3 Porous gravel plugged with LCM
Fig. 3–4 Natural horizontal fracture plugged with LCM
Fig. 3–5 Wide natural fracture sealed using cement

therefore are more apt to contact the bottom and top of the fracture and stay around the well bore. Some soft plugs are water reactive. These can be used where water is flowing in the fractures to react with the water and form M (water) plus DOB or DOB2C out of the water that is flowing. The volume of water flowing must be estimated and the optimum amounts of DOB and DOB2C mixed with it. If done objectively, water can be turned into a highly gelled cement that will set.

16

When the width of the natural fracture exceeds 1 foot (2 feet is probably the absolute maximum), it is probably more astute to drill blindly or with aerated mud and set pipe.

Induced Vertical Fractures*

Against an induced vertical fracture in a well in Louisiana, two 2,000-sack batches of neat portland cement were applied. After each application, the well was still on vacuum. Next, a 50-sack batch of FormAPlug, a surface-mixed soft plug (no longer manufactured), was applied. A squeeze pressure of 1,500 psi was developed and circulation regained. Why this spectacular difference in performance between neat cement slurries and the soft plugs?

In 1976 to 1977, a study was undertaken at Mobil Research and Development Corporation's Field Research Laboratory in Dallas to investigate the proper application of diesel oil, bentonite, and cement as lost-circulation materials. The basis for the study was that these materials are relatively cheap and are always at rigs. Also, the materials had shown considerable promise as lost-circulation materials. It was thought that if they could be fully understood and applied completely right, their performance could be vastly improved. In pursuit of this objective, the soft plug apparatus shown schematically in Fig. 3–6 was designed and built. Using the apparatus, mud (M) plus diesel oil-bentonite-two cement (DOB2C) could be mixed downhole (simulated) to form M+DOB2C and could be placed into a simulated induced vertical fracture by Bradenhead squeeze.

The simulated induced vertical fracture consisted of two sheets of plexiglass 4 ft in diameter. Bolts were run through the sheets as shown in Fig. 3–6 by the numbers 1–12. Springs were placed on the bolts so overburden could be simulated by tightening down on the bolts and compressing the springs. Run length was the time it took for the M+DOB2C to completely compress the inner row of springs or for the softer M+DOB2Cs to run out of the edges of the plexiglass.

For testing and comparing soft plugs, the apparatus was more simulation than required. After each run, the apparatus had to be dismantled, the samples taken for tests, and then reassembled. The procedure was laborious and time consuming. It was found that as reproducible, if not more reproducible results, could be obtained with

---

*All vertical fractures are induced. A natural vertical fracture will not take mud until it is opened or widened; it thereby becomes an induced fracture. While an induced fracture doesn't exist until it's induced, it's exactly like a natural vertical fracture once it is. That is, it widens and closes according to the pressures put upon it.

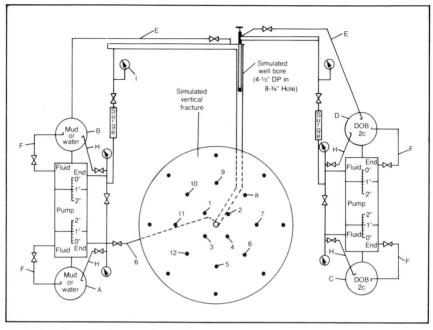

Fig. 3–6   Schematic diagram of soft-plug apparatus

considerably less effort by mixing the mud and diesel oil-bentonite-two cement in the desired proportions using a stirrer, pouring the mix out on a bench top, and kneading them together with a spatula.

Is it to be concluded, then, that the soft plug apparatus was a useless expenditure of funds? Definitely not! Using it, the means and mechanism by which induced vertical fractures must be plugged was demonstrated in the laboratory for the first time.

The mixing and Bradenhead squeezing of a 1:1½ M+DOB2C into the simulated fracture is shown in plates 3–1, 2, and 3. Note that at the start (1) there is no widening of the fracture. But as the M+DOB2C begins to form (2) a visible plug that is widening the fracture and compressing the springs forms at the center. The diesel oil, released in the process, can be seen extending beyond the plug. Finally (3), the M+DOB2C near the simulated well bore has completely compressed the springs of the inner row of bolts and a positive pressure of about 200 psi has developed. Any more mixing would have ruptured the plexiglass rather than extend the fracture. While there is 200 psi at the center, the outer edge of the fracture is open to the atmosphere. This proves beyond any doubt the mechanism for plugging induced vertical fractures.

Neat Portland cement slurries, even though they set hard, are not effective against induced vertical fractures. Soft plugs, also called plastic or soft cements, such as M+DOB, M+DOB2C, Bengum, Polymer Plug, or Flo-Chek, are effective. The reason for this is that the high gel strength of the soft plug causes it to resist flow into the fracture. This does two things: 1) it pries the fracture apart making it successively more difficult to pry it apart farther, and 2) it prevents the fracture propagation pressure from reaching the leading edge of the fracture and extending it. To make the seal permanent, something further is required. This is, once the induced vertical fracture has been pried apart, the fracture must be held apart while the lost circulation material either sets, dehydrates, or just loses mud. A neat Portland cement slurry placed on vacuum neither pries the fracture apart nor holds it apart until the cement sets.

Plugging Induced Vertical Fractures Using Bridging Agents

Induced vertical fractures can occur in any type formation but most often occur in shales or other nonporous formations. To plug such a fracture using bridging agents and do it permanently, the fracture must be permanently pried apart by packing it with dehydrated mud solids and bridging materials. Note that dehydration can only occur down the fracture because the fracture is in a nonporous formation. Several techniques call for developing and holding a gentle squeeze pressure on the bridging agent plug for ½ to 1 hour. Obviously, the purpose of this is to pack the widened fractures with LCM materials, thereby holding them apart and making the seal permanent.

Plugging Induced Vertical Fractures Using Portland Cements

Earlier, it was stated that neat Portland cement slurries were ineffective for sealing induced vertical fractures. This is absolutely true if the cement slurry is placed on vacuum; the hole does not fill nor does a squeeze pressure develop. For such a cement slurry to be effective, the fracture must be pried apart by developing squeeze pressure and held apart while the cement slurry dehydrates and then sets. There are two circumstances where it is possible to develop a squeeze pressure on an induced vertical fracture using portland cement slurries. The most obvious is when the fracture is in a porous formation (Fig. 3–9). This allows the cement slurry to dehydrate into the porous formation and to pry the fracture apart with dehydrated cement solids which then set.

The other situation is where, even though the formation is non-porous, a bridge can be formed at the leading edge of the fracture which allows dehydration down the fracture (Fig. 3–10). In some for-

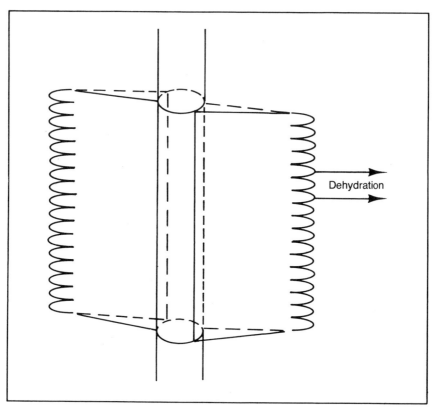

Fig. 3–7   Induced vertical fracture

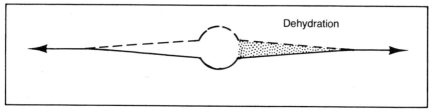

Fig. 3–8   Cross section of induced vertical fracture

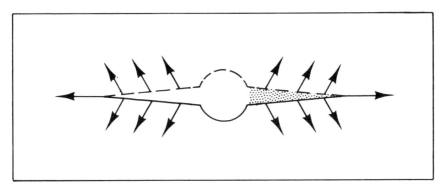

Fig. 3–9 Portland cement slurry against induced vertical fractures in a porous formation (cross section)

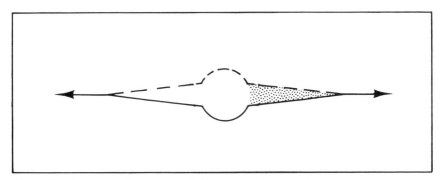

Fig. 3–10 Neat portland cement plus bridging agent (cross section)

mations, such a bridge can be initiated by adding a bridging agent such as 10–20 mesh frac sand (or other granular bridging agents) to the cement slurries. The cement slurry would then have two favorable properties: high filter loss (it completely dehydrates in two minutes) and bridging capability. Sound squeeze-cementing procedures are absolutely necessary for success.

Plugging Induced Vertical Fractures Using Soft Plugs

Soft plugs are very effective in sealing induced vertical fractures. Both M+DOB2C and M+DOB form a highly gelled mass when first mixed, which pries the fracture apart. But M+DOB2C then develops compressive strength (sets) to hold the fracture apart and make the seal permanent (Fig. 3–11). In the past 10 years, the author has not experienced a single failure with M+DOB2C when these placement conditions have been met.

21

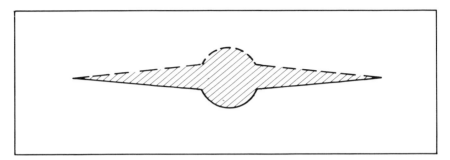

Fig. 3–11   M+DOB2C seal set in an induced vertical fracture

Since M+DOB never sets hard, it can deform to remake a seal in case the fracture is opened slightly. Further, as any soft plug is applied, squeeze pressure builds up, sealing the widest fracture but subsequently forcing the soft plug into fractures less severe and smaller in size. Most conventional Portland cement slurries do not exhibit the amount of gel strength that soft plugs do. As a result, squeeze pressure does not build up unless the cement slurry is dehydrated in some way as are LCM in mud or high-filter-loss slurry squeeze.

These plugging mechanisms need to be kept clearly in mind when choosing the functionally correct lost circulation material and technique for a particular application.

CHAPTER 4
Corrective Lost-Circulation Measures

In order to best apply curative techniques, the loss zone must be appraised in terms of location, type, and severity. Once this is accurately done, the lost circulation technique must be matched functionally and quickly to the severity of the loss zone.

Appraising the Zone

Even though they are mostly so reported, with the exception of the point of first loss, loss zones are usually not at the bit depth. Nine times out of ten, they recur at the point of first loss where the loss zone was sealed but reopened as drilling proceeded. The point of first loss usually occurs within 200–300 feet of the last casing shoe. However, the bit depth at every successive recurrence of the first loss will be logged as a new loss horizon. This has resulted in logging many loss zones at the bit that are up the hole at the point of first loss. If the loss is not found at the point of first loss or within 200–300 feet of the last casing shoe, it should then be found by temperature survey or by gamma-ray log and radioactive material. Evidence of where the loss zone is can also be obtained from how the lost-circulation materials performed and where they were found in the hole. As a matter of fact, the lost-circulation materials first applied might be chosen to some extent on how much they might reveal of where the loss zone is and if there are any complications. For example, a cement slurry will shed some light on where and how severe the zone is depending on whether it went up or down the hole, stayed put, or disappeared.

The type of loss zone is best determined from lithology, remembering that loss zones are horizontal to depths of 2,500–4,000 ft and vertical below these depths.

The severity of the loss zone is best determined by the amount of loss and the static mud column height. The static mud column height can be determined by running a piece of wood (4-foot long 4×4) on a wire line.

Correlating Technique to Severity

Loss zones can be classified as (a) seeping losses, (b) partial losses, (c) complete losses (hole full to fluid level at 200–500 ft), (d) complete losses (fluid level at 500–1,000 ft with evidence of long honeycomb sections and caverns), (e) partial or complete losses to deep induced vertical fractures, and (f) complete losses during underground blowouts.

Potential loss zones have first been placed into two broad classifications: horizontal and vertical. In general, loss zones lie horizontally above 2,500–4,000 ft and are vertical below these depths. The types of horizontal loss zones are porous sands and gravels, small to large natural fractures, and caverns. The types of vertical loss zones are induced fractures (natural vertical fractures must open to take mud and therefore become induced) and underground blowouts to induced vertical fractures.

Seeping losses can occur to any type loss zone in any type formation when the lost circulation agents in the mud are not fine enough to complete the seal. *Partial losses* occur in gravels, small natural horizontal fractures, and barely opened induced vertical fractures. *Complete losses* occur to long, open sections of gravel, long intervals of small natural horizontal fractures, large natural horizontal fractures, and partially opened induced vertical fractures. Severe complete losses occur to large, open natural horizontal fractures and caverns and to widely opened induced vertical fractures.*

Matching the Cure to Zone Severity

A correlation of the lost-circulation technique that should succeed most economically with the type and severity of the loss zones is given in Table 4–1. This approach to the control of lost circulation has been to assess the severity of the lost-circulation zone and then match the remedial material and technique to it in terms of both size and function.

Before any conclusions are drawn or recommendations are made for use of bridging agents for curing mud losses, a brief review of the art is in order. The data, developed by Howard and Scott in Fig. 4–1, show the effect of concentration of lost circulation (bridging) materials when sealing fractures.[1] Up to a concentration of 20 lb/bbl, the size of the fracture sealed using bridging agents in mud (technique 2, Chapter 5) increases. But at 20 lb/bbl, the fracture size vs. material concentration curve becomes asmatotic to the fracture-size-sealed line. This

---

* The width to which an induced vertical fracture opens depends on the pressure deficiency between the formation it occurs in and that in the well bore. The greater the deficiency, the wider the fracture.

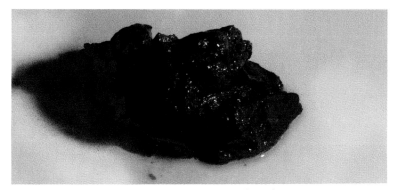

Plate 1.   Water + DOB2C (1:1)

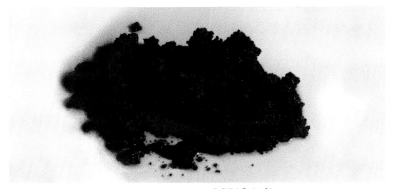

Plate 2.   Water + DOB2C (1:2)

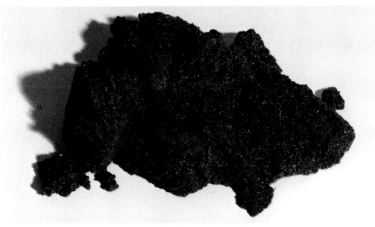

Plate 3.   Water + DOB2C (1:3)

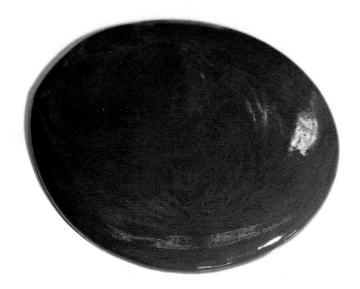

Plate 4. Mud + DOB2C (4:1)

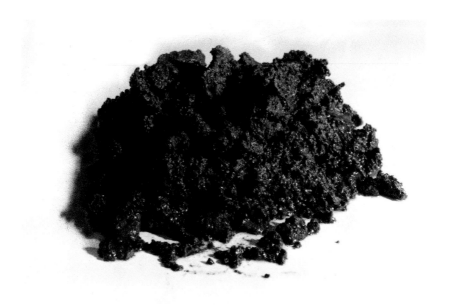

Plate 6. Mud + DOB2C (1:1)

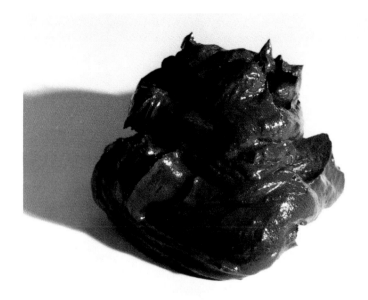

Plate 5.   Mud + DOB2C (3:1)

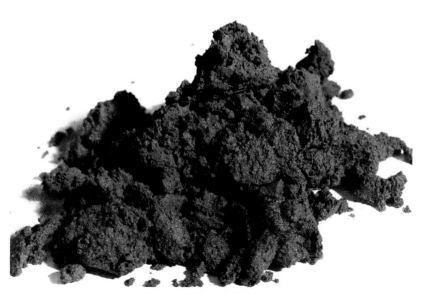

Plate 7.   Mud + DOB2C (1:3)

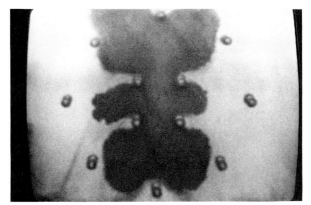

Plate 3-1

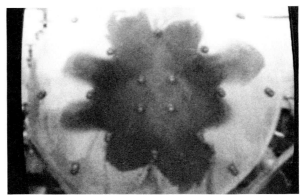

Plate 3-2

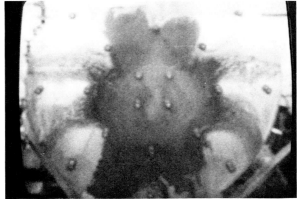

Plate 3-3

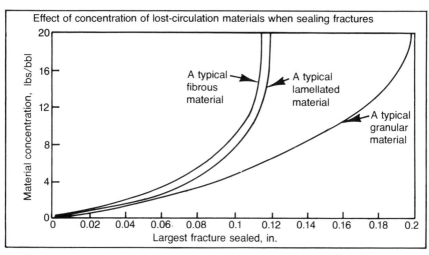

Fig. 4–1 Effect of concentration of lost-circulation materials when sealing fractures (after Howard and Scott)

Summary of material evaluation tests				
Material	Type	Description	Concentration lbs/bbl	Largest fracture sealed, in. 0 0.04 0.08 0.12 0.16 0.20
Nut shell	Granular	50% 3/16 +10 mesh 50% 10 +100 mesh	20	
Plastic	Granular	,,	20	
Limestone	Granular	,,	40	
Sulfur	Granular	,,	120	
Nut shell	Granular	50% 10 +16 mesh 50% 10 +100 mesh	20	
Expanded perlite	Granular	50% 3/16 +10 mesh 50% 10 + 100 mesh	60	
Cellophane	Lamellated	¾ in. flakes	8	
Sawdust	Fibrous	¼ in. particles	10	
Prairie hay	Fibrous	½ in. fibers	10	
Bark	Fibrous	¾ in. fibers	10	
Cotton seed hulls	Granular	Fine	10	
Prairie hay	Fibrous	¾ in. particles	12	
Cellophane	Lamellated	½ in. flakes	8	
Shredded wood	Fibrous	¼ in. fibers	8	
Sawdust	Fibrous	1/16 in. particles	20	

Fig. 4–2 Summary of material evaluation tests (after Howard and Scott)

25

TABLE 4–1 Match the Lost Circulation Remedial Technique Functionally to the Severity of the Loss Zone

Type of loss	Severity of loss, bbl/hr	Loss zone geometry	Lost circulation remedial technique	Effective in WBM	OBM*
Seeping	1–10	to Horizontal loss zones** to Induced vert. fractures	Technique 2—Plug of *fine* bridging agents in mud	yes	yes
			Technique 3—High-filter-loss slurry squeeze with *fine* bridging agents	yes	yes
Partial	10–500	to Horizontal loss zones** to Induced vert. fractures	Technique 1—Pull up and wait (primarily for induced vert. frac)	yes	partial
			Technique 2—Plug of *medium* bridging agents in mud	yes	yes
			Technique 3—High-filter-loss slurry squeeze with *fine* bridging agents	yes	yes
Complete	500–complete	to Horizontal loss zones**	Technique 3—High-filter-loss slurry squeeze with coarse bridging agents	yes	yes
			Technique 4B—Thixotropic cement (for other choices, see Chapter 5)	yes	no
			Technique 5—Mud + diesel-oil-bentonite-two cement (M+DOB2C)	yes	no
			Technique 7—Downhole-mixed soft plug (mud-diesel oil-bentonite, (M+DOB) (for other choices, see Chapter 5)	yes	yes
			Technique 7D—Downhole-mixed soft plug (sodium silicate, calcium chloride, cement squeeze Flow-Chek)	yes	yes
Long honeycomb or caverns; only in limestones	Complete	to Horizontal loss zones**	Technique 3—High-filter-loss slurry squeeze with 25–35 lb/bbl of coarse bridging agents	yes	yes
			Technique 5—Downhole-mixed soft/hard plug continuously mixed in large amounts of M+DOB2C	yes	no
			Technique 9—Drill blind or with aerated mud and set pipe	yes	yes

Loss zone	Severity	Formation/mud	Corrective technique		
Deep induced fractures	Complete	Vertical in WBM or OBM	Technique 1—Pull up and wait	yes	partial
		in WBM	Technique 5—Downhole-mixed soft/hard plug (M+DOB2C)	yes	no
		in WBM	Technique 7—Downhole-mixed soft plug (M+DOB) (for other choices, see Chapter 5)	yes	no
		in WBM	Technique 7D—Downhole-mixed soft plug (sodium silicate, calcium chloride, cement squeeze, Flo-Chek)	yes	yes
		in OBM	Technique 3—High-filter-loss slurry squeeze with coarse bridging agents	yes	yes
		in OBM	Technique 4A—Neat portland cement	yes	yes
		in OBM	Technique 7D—Downhole-mixed soft plug (sodium silicate, calcium chloride, cement squeeze, Flo-Chek)	yes	yes
Underground blowout	Complete	Induced in WBM	Technique 5—Downhole-mixed soft/hard plug (M+DOB2C)	yes	no
		Vertical fracture in WBM	Control with barite plug; repair loss zone using technique 5 or run pipe	yes	yes
		in OBM	Control with barite plug; repair loss zone using technique 7D or run pipe	yes	yes

*Usually not in use where loss zones are horizontal
**Consist of porous sands and gravels, natural fractures, and honeycomb and caverns
WBM—water-base mud
OBM—oil-base mud

shows that the largest fracture sealed also depends on the largest particles in the bridging agent. A typical ¼-inch fibrous material (sawdust) would plug an 0.11-inch fracture; a typical ¾-inch flake material (cellophane) would seal a 0.12-inch fracture; and a typical ³⁄₁₆-inch granular material (nut shell) would seal a 0.20-inch fracture. The data in Fig. 4–2 further demonstrate the relationship between the largest particles the bridging agent contains and the largest fracture it would seal.

It can be concluded from this that both the size of the bridging agent and its concentration in the mud determine the largest fracture it will seal. Of these, size is the more important. For a bridging agent to be effective in sealing a loss zone, it must contain some particles that approximate the width of the loss zone in size. It follows that the size of the bridging agent must be matched to the severity (width) of the loss zone.

Glenn and Jenkins (1951) tested ground leather (Leather Floc) as a bridging material.[2] Partial results of their study, shown in Fig. 4–3, def-

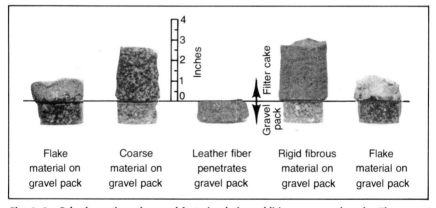

Fig. 4–3 Cake formation of several lost-circulation additives on gravel packs. The center item shows how the leather fiber penetrates the gravel beds approximately one inch. The other materials merely accumulate on top of the gravel pack.

initely proved that Leather Floc was functionally different from other fibers in that it penetrated the gravel pack, binding the gravel together instead of collecting on top of the gravel pack as flake and coarser, more rigid fibers did. The results definitely proved that Leather Floc, if present in a blend of bridging agents, would assist in forming an in-formation seal that was more permanent than one just resting on the face of the gravel.

Wilson (1955) demonstrated that a 2-component blend of a granular bridging agent (sawdust or rice hulls) and a fibrous bridging agent (Leather Floc) were more effective in sealing a simulated loss zone than either material alone.[3,4] This was the first published evidence that blends of bridging agents (granular, fiber, and flake) would outperform any one of them alone.

Howard and Scott designed and built their own test apparatus for bridging agents. However, independent testing of bridging agents throughout the industry became more and more prevalent. In 1961, the API Standardization Committee organized a task group to develop an API standard procedure to test bridging agents. First, test procedures of 12 companies were surveyed. Next, samples of bridging agents were distributed to 11 companies that ran tests using their own test muds and apparatus. "API RP 13B: Standard Procedure for Testing Drilling Fluids; Section 10—Bridging Materials for Regaining Circulation" grew out of this work. (See Appendix A.)

Using API test procedures, Lummus ran a series of tests of bridging agents designed to produce a marketable one-sack blend that would be effective against gravels, vugs, and induced and natural fractures.[5,6] First he chose 10 commercially available products (Table 4–2) that possessed desirable properties. API tests of the 10 materials showed all would seal slots of from 0.06 inch to 0.13 inch, none would pass the 1,000-psi marble test, and three would pass the 1,000-psi BB shot test. The three that sealed the BBs were either fibers or flake.

As one of his objectives, Lummus wanted to develop a single package of bridging agents that would be effective in sealing both the horizontal and vertical loss zone. He concluded from his preliminary tests that it must be a blend of granular, fiber, and flake bridging agents. The results of some of his tests on such blends appear in Tables 4–2 and 4–3. The various components of the blends were added in equal proportions. Finally, a most effective blend of bridging agents emerged from the test data. It consisted of amounts of four components in equal proportions:

1. Granular—coarse-to-medium walnut shells
2. Fiber—coarse-to-medium cane fibers
3. Fiber—fine nylon carpet fibers
4. Flake—medium to large (¼-inch) cellophane

The data in Table 4–3 show that 30–40 lb/bbl of the above blend (tradenamed Kwik Seal) would seal a 0.20-inch slot. Kwik Seal was made available commercially in October 1965. By October 1966, it had been used in 200 wells in varied areas with above-average success.

Kwik Seal is available in a coarse, medium, and fine grind for several reasons. First, as this author preaches, the size of the bridging agent must be matched to the severity of the loss zone. Coarse materials would just go by a seeping loss without any entering it; fine materials would not seal a ¼-inch induced vertical fracture. Second,

TABLE 4–2 Examples of Results Obtained Using Statistical Program Design. All Tests Conducted Using 10 lb/bbl Total Concentrations; Additives Mixed in Equal Proportions.

Mixture	Slot Size Sealed at 100 psi		Total Volume ÷ Slot Size, cc/in.		Atmospheric Volume ÷ Slot Size, cc/in.		Seal Pressure × Slot Size, lbs/in.	
	Observed	Computed	Observed	Computed	Observed	Computed	Observed	Computed
1. Nutshell granules (Medium) cellophane flakes carpet fibers	0.20 in.	0.12	2450	1877	500	646	10.0	3.4
2. Nutshell granules (Medium) plastic granules (Medium) cellophane flakes leather fibers	0.08	0.08	313	2097	0	95	0.8	1.8
3. Nutshell granules (Medium) mica flakes carpet fibers ground tire cord	0.08	0.11	1875	2115	63	806	1.2	2.3
4. Nutshell granules (Coarse) plastic granules (Medium) mica flakes cane fiber and pulp	0.08	0.13	3125	2613	125	764	0.8	3.4
5. Nutshell granules (Coarse) laminated plastic cellophane flakes cane fiber and pulp	0.20	0.17	950	2276	500	589	5.0	3.7

TABLE 4–3 Performance of Various Concentrations of Mixed Sealing Material in Mud

		Static shot test	Static marble-bed test		BB shot-bed test	
	Largest	Volume through at	Volume through at		Volume through at	
Concentration lb/bbl	Slot sealed inches	1,000 psi ml	1,000 psi ml	Seal	1,000 psi ml	Seal
10	0.10	500	All	no	1,700	Yes
20	0.13	250	1,900	yes	2,050	Yes
30	0.16	400	1,700	yes	800	Yes
40	0.20	300	1,700	yes	1,800	Yes

Mixed sealing material composed of: coarse-to-medium walnut shells, coarse-to-medium cane fibers, nylon fibers, and medium-to-large (1-in.) cellophane flake (after Lummus).

coarse materials would immediately plug standard $\frac{9}{32}$-inch jet bit nozzles. Medium and fine Kwik Seal would not plug a $\frac{9}{32}$-inch nozzle. But the data in Table 4–4 show that the size of the fracture plugged decreases by half if medium is used instead of coarse.

Obviously, the drilling industry is not going to apply Kwik Seal, even though it fills a need and has performed well, to the exclusion of all the other bridging agents available because there are circumstances where a single bridging agent might be more effective and cheaper.[7] Again, a blend higher in large-sized granular agent should be run in a high-filter-loss slurry.

TABLE 4–4 Comparison of Coarse and Medium Grinds of Mixed Sealing Material in Mud (after Lummus)

Test	30 lb/bbl Coarse-grind material	30 lb/bbl Medium-grind material
1. Pumping test through 9/32 in. standard jet bit nozzles	Plugged immediately	Flowed through at 200 psi
2. Static slot		
Largest slot sealed, in.	0.16	0.08
Total vol through, ml	400	100
3. Dynamic slot:		
Largest slot sealed, in.	0.13	0.06
Total vol through, ml	600	0.50
4. Static marble bed:		
Vol through at 100 psi, ml	500	400
Vol through at 1000 psi, ml	1,700	1,200
5. BB-shot bed:		
Vol through at 100 psi, ml	400	300
Vol through at 1000 psi, ml	800	800

Therefore, when bridging agents have application, an effective mixture should best contain at least two components: granular and fibrous agents. A useful three-component mixture is 1–6 parts granular (nut shells), two parts coarse-to-fine fiber (cane, nylon, flax, asbestos, leather), and one part flake (cellophane).

The size of the bridging agent should be matched to the severity of the loss zone. Little advantage is gained if the concentration of lost-circulation materials in a mud system or high-filter-loss slurry exceeds 15–20 lb/bbl (see Fig. 4–1); pump trouble and poor mud properties may result from higher concentrations. It is important to increase the size and the amount of the granular agent if conventionally sized agents are not effective. If bridging agents are to be applied in a slug of mud (technique 2), then concentrations up to 30–40 lb/bbl can be more effective.

Bridging agents can be safely added to both oil- and water-base muds. However, they are more effective in water-base muds because the filter loss is higher, allowing more dehydration and better widening and packing of the loss zone. Another reason that bridging agents have a narrower use in oil muds is that oil muds are normally not used at shallow depths where loss zones are horizontal. Bridging agents might be better carried in oil-base spacers that usually are prepared without the filter-loss control agent and thus have a higher filter loss. This has not been tried.

Mud losses, ranging in severity from seeps to complete losses into ⅛-inch to ¼-inch natural and induced fractures, can be stopped using bridging agents. For the agent to function, some of it must be the approximate size of the opening to be plugged. Accordingly, fine granular material (walnut shells, pecan shells, mica), fine fiber (leather, flax, nylon, carpet, cane, asbestos) and ½-inch to 1-inch cellophane flake should be used against seeping losses.

Coarse granular material (¼-inch or ½-inch walnut or pecan shells), coarse fiber (shredded hard wood or cedar), medium fiber (shredded redwood or sugar cane), fine fiber (leather, flax, nylon or asbestos), and coarse flake (1-inch cellophane flake) should be used against complete losses. Note that as the severity of the loss zone increases, only the size of the bridging agent is increased, not the concentration (Table 4–1).

With the bridging agents available today that can be applied through mud pumps, mud losses to natural and induced fractures up to ¼-inch in width can be plugged. A recent report indicates that beer bottles have been successfully applied to a severe loss zone as bridging agents directly downhole. Most rigid hollow objects filled with drilling fluid or a lighter liquid would be strong enough yet have a density near that of mud, making it possible for the flow of the mud to carry them intact to restrictions in the loss zone.

When the width of a natural fracture or cavern exceeds this size, cement (technique 4) or soft-plug techniques (techniques 5, 6, and 7) should be used. If applied correctly, cements that set hard should plug natural horizontal fractures and caverns ¼ inch to 1 foot in width. Two-foot fractures are the absolute upper limit. Caverns larger than this should be drilled blind or with aerated mud and pipe set (technique 9).

Cement slurries that set hard and have low gel strength (technique 4) are not effective against natural and induced vertical fractures. Soft plugs, also called plastic and soft cements (technique 5, M+DOB2C; technique 6, Pal-mix 110R; technique 7, M+DOB, Bengum, Polymer Plug, OM+WOB, Flo-chek) are effective. This is because the high gel strength of the plastic cement causes it to resist flow into the fracture, opening the fracture and making it increasingly more difficult to pry it apart farther. Also it prevents propagation pressure from reaching the end of the fracture and extending it. NOTE: The author has never experienced a failure where it was possible to develop a squeeze pressure on the loss zone and then hold the pressure until the cement set.

Usual Causes of Failure to Cure

Some of the most usual causes—directly or indirectly—for failure to cure loss of circulation are as follows:

1) The location of the loss zone is often not established, resulting in placing the materials in the wrong place. Many loss zones logged at the bit are actually up the hole at the first point of loss. Lost circulation zones are usually not on bottom (at bit depth) but are near the last casing depth or the point of first loss.

2) Lost-circulation materials and techniques are not systematically matched to the type and severity of the loss zone.

3) Many times there is a reluctance to proceed rapidly to the technique required to match the severity of the loss zone (drill blind and set pipe).

4) Adequate records are not kept that describe the losses and the materials and techniques effective against them. Accurate accounts of the experience in an area are valuable.

5) In cementing, the columns are not balanced and drilling mud breaks through the plug before it sets. In addition, when the pipe is withdrawn from the hole after placement, the mud level in the annulus

decreases and the mud from the formation can break through the freshly placed slurry. Balanced column, dropping the plug and spot across, pull up, and squeeze techniques should be employed (see technique 4).

To increase the success ratio, the lost-circulation materials and techniques must be functionally related to the losses they cure without delay. For example, where a reasonable amount (say 15–20 lb/bbl) of bridging material has not worked in a high-filter-loss slurry squeeze, it is usually useless to apply higher concentrations of the same materials. The next step should be to increase the size of the granular bridging material. If this does not succeed, then a more severe technique is probably required (cements or soft plugs).

It cannot be stressed too strongly that the lost-circulation technique must be matched to the severity of the loss zone without delay.

CHAPTER 5
Lost-Circulation Materials and Techniques

On several occasions, I was asked to recommend lost-circulation materials and techniques for remote drilling sites. The following materials were recommended:

1) Coarse, medium and fine granular, fiber, and flake bridging agents. These could come as a blend of granular, fiber, and flake agents or be separately packaged.

2) Diesel oil, bentonite, cement, barite, and a dispersant, filter loss agent and retarder for the cement and thinners for the barite plugs were always supplied; the amounts were just increased accordingly. Some will say that this selection of materials is woefully inadequate; however, seven of the nine lost-circulation techniques and both barite plugs used these materials (asterisked).

*Technique 1—Pull up and wait
*Technique 2—Bridging agents in mud—either in water- or oil-base muds
*Technique 3—High-filter-loss slurry squeeze with and without cement
*Technique 4—Portland cement—neat or plus additives
*Technique 5—Downhole-mixed soft/hard plugs (DOB2C)
 Technique 6—Surface-mixed soft plugs (not available)
*Technique 7—Downhole-mixed soft plugs (DOB)
 Technique 8—Specialized agents (not available)
*Technique 9—Drill blind or with aerated mud and set pipe
*Barite and barite-in-oil plugs

Actually, my job included troubleshooting severe lost circulation problems. Because I never visited a location where bridging agents would succeed, I have had very little direct experience in applying them. Most of my expertise with bridging agents is borrowed. My direct experience is with loss zones that bridging agents and other conventional materials had failed to seal.

In view of a 100% success rate, I believe that if the above materials are applied correctly, they will cure any loss zone that can be cured. Be assured, however, that I will recommend and use any other product available in the drilling industry today that is (a) lower in cost, (b) as available, (c) a better performer, or (d) is especially applicable where oil muds are in use.

Technique 1—Pull Up and Wait

Use this technique against seeping, partial, and complete losses to induced vertical fractures. The mechanism by which this works is that the fracture was created by inadvertantly putting excessive but unrequired pressure on the formation. If the pressure is removed, the fracture, given time, will close and heal. Horizontal loss zones—gravels, natural fractures, vugs, honeycombs, and caverns—do not close and heal in this manner because they are not induced but occur naturally with the overburden being self-supporting.

At the first indication of loss to an induced vertical fracture, drilling and circulation should be stopped. The bit should be pulled to a point of safety and the hole permitted to remain quiet for a period of 4 to 8 hours. After such a waiting period, good drilling techniques must be followed in getting back to bottom to keep minimum pressures on the formations.

Speculating that returns will not be obtained by waiting, a 100-bbl plug of bridging agents in mud or a similar volume of high-filter-loss slurry can be mixed during the waiting period.

Where water-base minds are in use, half of the losses in the Gulf Coast area were corrected in this manner.[8] Surprisingly, once the fracture had healed, it would support virtually the same pressure as before being fractured. This technique is not as effective where oil muds are in use. For example, in a well being drilled under the Mediterranean Sea, a formation that held 14.0 ppg mud equivalent at the shoe of the 20-inch casing would hold only a 11.5 mud equivalent after being fractured with invert mud under a mud ring. To get back the required formation strength, 16-inch casing had to be run at a cost over $1 million.

When drilling with oil mud, drilling people should not depend on an induced fracture to close and heal. They should take every reasonable precaution to avoid fracturing the formation.

Technique 2—Plug of Bridging Agents in Mud (Water and Oil Base)

Use this technique from Lummus against seeping and partial losses and less-severe complete losses to both horizontal and vertical loss zones. A plug of bridging agents in mud is mixed and applied as follows:

1) Establish the approximate point of loss, type of formation taking the mud, height the mud stands in the hole, and rate of loss. If a vertical fracture of the formation due to a pressure surge is suspected, the most probable point of loss is just below the casing shoe.

2) Use open-ended drillpipe for placing the plug if practical. Otherwise, use open watercourse bits or jet bits with nozzles removed. If materials must be placed through a jet bit, medium-to-fine-sized bridging agents should be used to prevent plugging the bit.

3) Mix a 100 to 500-bbl plug of bridging agents in mud. A mixture of coarse, medium, and fine granular, fiber, and flake bridging agents is available and could be substituted for those added separately. First, add 10–20 lb/bbl of bentonite to 80 bbl of water that has been pretreated with ½ lb/bbl of sodium carbonate and ¼ lb/bbl caustic soda to remove calcium and sodium ions. Allow the bentonite to yield. Add ½ lb/bbl lime.

Next, add 15 lb/bbl of coarse walnut or pecan shells. Other coarse granular agents (ground peach or olive pits, phenoseal, almond shells or sawdust) can be substituted if the nut shells are not available. Finally, add 5 lb/bbl coarse-medium fibers (wood or cane). Add 5 lb/bbl of medium-to-fine fibers (wood, cane, nylon, flax). Add 5 lb/bbl of 1-inch cellophane flake.

Note: The size of the bridging agent should be tailored to the severity of the loss and to the size of the mud courses of the bit. The filter loss of the slurry should be lowered only to prevent the hole from sloughing; the mud density should be raised to the point required to control the well. Actually, the bridging agents can be added directly to the water-base mud in use at the time of the circulation loss.

4) Place the plug through open-ended drillpipe opposite the loss zone. Pump at 1 bbl/min until the materials have stopped the loss. Repeat once more if the hole does not fill and then proceed to technique 3, high-filter-loss slurry squeeze, if there is still no indication of success. If the hole fills, close the blowout preventers (rams) and, with a mud gun open, squeeze the annulus with 50 psi for 30 min. Measure the pressure on the annulus using a 0–300-psi gauge.

5) If circulation is established and a low-solids mud is in use, screen out the bridging agents immediately.

Technique 2A—Pronto Plug

Pronto Plug is a blend of water-soluble polymers and sized, dehydrated, sterile, hardwood particles. Use it against mud losses to shallow horizontal loss zones such as vuggy and fractured limestone, gravel beds, and shell reefs. The hardwood particles are a bridging agent and also adsorb water to help dehydrate the slurry once it's in place. A Pronto Plug can be complexed into a semiplastic mass.

Normally, the plug is mixed by adding 1 sack (40 lb) of Pronto Plug per bbl of mix water or brine. If the plug is weighted or treated with additional bridging agent, as little as ¼ sk/bbl may be required.

Bridging agents can be run in a slug of oil mud, also. The procedure for applying the slug of bridging agents in oil mud is the same as for bridging agents in mud. Some care must be exercised to avoid bridging agents that are water-wet, thereby lowering the stability of inverted emulsion muds.

In *World Oil's* 1980–1981 "Guide to Drilling, Workover and Completion Fluids," a list of all the bridging agents in use is given.[7] All have application in water-base muds; some have application in both water-base muds, inverted-emulsion muds, and full oil-base muds. The list has been carefully reviewed and the bridging agents with application in both water and oil base muds selected. The agents, according to the listing, that can be used to prepare bridging agents in a slug of oil mud are shown below.

Granular: ground nut hulls (walnuts, peach pits, almonds, olive pits, pecans), laminated plastic, calcium carbonate, barite, ground coal, ground neoprene, and expanded perlite.

Fiber: Cane, shredded redwood and cedar, leather, asbestos, cottonseed hulls, and pig hair.

Flake: Cellophane, wood shavings, and mica.

Proportions of these materials would be three parts granular, two parts fiber, and one part flake. The compatibility of all bridging agents with the oil-phase mud in which they are to be used should be reviewed before they are applied.

Technique 3—High-Filter-Loss Slurry Squeezes (HFLSS)[9, 10, 11]

Use this technique against seeping and partial losses and less severe complete losses to both horizontal and vertical loss zones. There are slight differences in application to these zones, but the main distinction is increasing the size of the bridging agent as the loss zone becomes more severe. Next, the approximate point of loss should be established and the type of formation taking mud defined. If an induced vertical fracture of the formation due to pressure is suspected, the most probable point of loss is just below the casing shoe.

Seeping Loss

1) Mix 100 bbl of slurry. Add 16–20 lb/bbl of attapulgite or sepiolite clay to 80 bbl of water. (Sepiolite clay behaves similarly to attapulgite clay in salt water.) If these clays are not available, use 5–20 lb/bbl bentonite and pretreat the water with ¼ lb/bbl sodium and ¼ lb/bbl caustic soda to remove calcium and magnesium ions. Allow the clay to yield.

Then add ½ lb/bbl lime and 50 lb/bbl diatomaceous-earth materials (Diacel D, Diaseal M, or a suitable substitute such as powdered limestone.) Diaseal M is a mixture of diatomaceous earth and fine asbestos fibers (Flosal or Visbestos). If this mixture is used, attapulgite is not required. Diacel D, Diacel M, and Flosal are marketed by Drilling Specialities. Visbestos is marketed by Montello, Inc. Another source of diatomaceous earth is Litepoz 2, marketed by Dowell.

Next, add 5 lb/bbl of fine mica, 5 lb/bbl fine walnut or almond shells, 4 lb/bbl medium to fine fiber, and 1 lb/bbl shredded leather.

2) Set the bit at the top of or opposite the loss zone. Displace the slurry to the end of the drillpipe.

3) Close the rams; leave a mud gun open to control squeeze pressure. Gently squeeze (50 psi maximum) material into the loss zone at a rate of 1 bbl/min. Gradually shut the gun and hold the squeeze pressure 4–8 hr or until it dissipates. Measure the squeeze pressure on the annulus using a 0–300-psi gauge.

To avoid fracturing other zones, safe squeeze pressures in excess of mud-hydrostatic pressure should be used. For example:

0–1,000 ft: 0–200 psi squeeze pressure

1,000–5,000 ft: 100–500 psi squeeze pressure

5,000–ft and deeper: 500 psi squeeze pressure

Surface pressure plus mud-column pressure should never exceed overburden pressure.

Partial Loss

1) Mix 100 bbl of slurry. Add 10–15 lb/bbl of attapulgite or sepiolite clay to 80 bbl of water. If these clays are not available, substitute bentonite and treat the water as before. Then add ½ lb/bbl lime and 50 lb/bbl diatomaceous earth materials (as before) or a suitable substitute (powdered limestone). Use barite only if the mud weight is 12 ppg or higher or if it is the only inert powdered material available.

Finally, add 8 lb/bbl of granular lost-circulation material (coarse walnuts, peach pits, or olive pits), 4 lb/bbl of medium wood or cane fiber, 1 lb/bbl of fine fiber (cane, paper, nylon, leather) and 3 lb/bbl of coarse cellophane flakes.

2) Set the drillpipe with the open end at the top of or opposite the loss zone.

3) Displace 25 bbl of slurry into the zone at a rate of 2–4 bbl/min.

4) Shut down for 20–30 min.

5) Displace another 25 bbl of slurry at the same rate.

6) Continue this procedure, alternately waiting and displacing until the hole fills. Sometimes two 100-bbl batches will be required. The drillpipe should be reciprocated during the operations to prevent it from sticking.

7) When the hole fills, close the rams and squeeze the annulus with 50–100 psi by displacing very slowly (1 bbl/min) down the drillpipe. A mud gun should be left open to control surges. Attach a 0–300-psi gauge to the annulus so that low pressure values can be easily read. Maintain the squeeze for 30–60 min.

8) Pull out of the hole, pick up a bit, and go back to drilling.

Complete Loss

The same technique is employed as that used for partial loss except the slurry composition is somewhat different.

1) Add 10–15 lb/bbl of attapulgite or sepiolite clay to 80 bbl of water. If these clays are not available, use bentonite and treat water as before. Add ½ lb/bbl lime and 50 lb/bbl diatomaceous earth materials (as before). Use barite only if the mud weight is 12 lb/gal or higher or if it is the only inert material available.

Add 8 lb/bbl of granular lost-circulation materials (coarse walnuts, peach pits, olive pits up to ¼-in to ½-in), 3 lb/bbl coarse-to-medium wood or cane fiber, 3 lb/bbl of medium-to-fine fiber (wood, cane, nylon, leather), and 3 lb/bbl of large cellophane flakes.

2) Set the drillpipe open end at the top of or opposite to the loss zone.

3) Displace 25 bbl of slurry into the zone at a rate of 2–4 bbl/min.

4) Shut down for 20 to 30 min.

5) Displace another 25 bbl of slurry at the same rate.

6) Continue this procedure, alternately waiting and displacing until the hole fills. Sometimes two 100-bbl batches will be required. The drillpipe should be reciprocated during these operations to keep it from sticking.

7) When the hole fills, close the rams and squeeze the annulus with 50–100 psi by displacing the slurry very slowly down the drillpipe. If the rig pumps are used for the squeeze, a mud gun should be left open to control surges. Attach a 0–300-psi pressure gauge to the annulus so that low pressure values can be easily read. Maintain the squeeze for 30–60 min.

8) Pull out of the hole, pick up the bit, and go back to drilling.

If there is no evidence of improvement after two batches, proceed to techniques 4, 5, 6, or 7.

Technique 3A—High-Water Loss, High-Solids Squeeze with Cement (HWL+HSwC)

In 1977, Cagle and Mathews disclosed the addition of portland cement to the conventional high-filter-loss slurry squeeze.[12,13] This incorporated possible functional improvement because, once the solids from the HFL+HSwC squeeze widen and pack the fracture by dehydrating, they then develop compressive strength (set) to make the seal more permanent. HWL+HSwC is used primarily for complete losses. (For seeping and partial losses the size of the bridging agents would be reduced to fine and medium, respectfully).

Where water-base muds are in use, I prefer to use technique 5 (M+DOB2C) over HFLSS or HWL+HSwC, which also have application, because it has been almost 100% effective. But because water-base mud is required to form it, M+DOB2C has little or no application where oil muds are in use. Therefore HFLSS or HWL+HSwC squeeze, which are surface mixed, have application where oil muds are in use.[14] Because of the above consideraions, the procedure for mixing and placing HWL+HSwC squeeze are presented where an oil-base mud is in use.

The following well parameters are assumed: 47-lb $9\frac{5}{8}$-inch casing is set at 10,000 feet; an $8\frac{1}{2}$-inch hole has been drilled to 11,000 feet using 5-in. drillpipe; the loss zone is an induced vertical fracture at 10,100 feet (within 300 feet f the shoe); and a 16.0 ppg Invermul mud is in use.

1) Fill the annulus with fresh water (It takes 64 bbl showing that the static fluid level was at 683 feet). Now there are 1,313 feet of water and 8.787 feet of 16.0 ppg mud in the annulus which calculates to an average column weight of 15.0 ppg. Mix the HWL-HSwC slurry at this weight.

2) To mix 100 bbl of correctly weighted HWL+HS$_w$C slurry, add 10–15 lb/bbl attapulgite or sepiolite clay to 65 bbl of fresh or sea water (Table 5–1). If these clays are not available, use 5–20 lb/bbl of bentonite

TABLE 5–1   Suggested Materials for a One-Barrel Mixture of an HWL+HS-cement
Squeeze* (after Cagle and Mathews)

Density, lb/gal	HWL+HS Additive, lb	Cement Sack		Barite Sack	Water Barrel
		(Min.)	(Max.)	(Average)	
9.5	15	1.0	1.4	0	0.84
10.0	20	1.0	1.4	0	0.83
11.0	20	1.0	1.4	1.0	0.78
12.0	20	1.0	1.4	1.4	0.75
13.0	20	1.0	1.4	1.8	0.72
14.0	20	1.0	1.4	2.5	0.68
15.0	15	1.0	1.3	2.7	0.65
16.0	15	1.0	1.2	3.8	0.57
17.0	12	1.0	1.2	3.8	0.57
18.0	10	1.0	1.0	4.4	0.54

*To prevent deviating the hole, the set strength of the dehydrated solids should not exceed 1,000-psi. All slurries contain 18 lb/bbl fiber and 3 lb/bbl flake. All slurries are to be retarded to the safe minimum thickening time and should be pumpable enough for easy mixing and placement.

and pretreat the fresh water, if required, with ¼ lb/bbl sodium carbonate and ¼ lb/bbl caustic soda to remove calcium and magnesium ions. Allow the clay to yield for 1 hour.

Then add ¼-lb/bbl lime and 10–25 lb/bbl of diatomaceous-earth materials (Diacel D, Diaseal M) or a suitable substitute such as powdered limestone. Diaseal M is a mixture of diatomaceous earth and fine asbestos fibers (Flosal or Visbestos). If Diaseal M is used, attapulgite or bentonite is not required and either fresh or sea water can be used without treatment. Use barite only if the mud weight is 12.0 lb/gal or higher or if there is no other inert filler available.

3) Add 9 lb/bbl of granular bridging agents (coarse walnuts, peach pits, olive pits, Phenoseal) up to ¼ inch to ½ inch in size, 3 lb/bbl coarse-to-medium wood or cane fiber, 3 lb/bbl of medium to fine fiber (wood, cane, nylon, leather) and 3 lb/bbl of large cellophane flake. Then add 270 100-lb sacks of barite and 65 94-lb sacks of cement (Table 5–1).

4) Set the drillpipe with the open end 100 feet above the shoe (9,900 feet).

5) Displace the HWL+HSwC slurry to the end of the drillpipe (Fig. 5–1). If there still are water returns, close the BOPs. Displace 50 bbl of slurry down hole and into the loss zone at a rate of 2–4 bbl/min. Do not attempt to place coarse bridging agents through a jet bit; they plug it immediately every time.

6) Shut down for 20–30 min.

7) Displace 25 bbl of slurry at the same rate.

8) Continue this procedure, alternately waiting and displacing, until the hole fills and a squeeze pressure develops (Fig. 5–2). Sometimes two 100-bbl batches will be required. The drillpipe, particularly if it's out in open hole, should be moved during these operations to prevent it from sticking.

9) When the hole fills or, as in this case, it stands full or flows, close the rams and squeeze with 200–500 psi by displacing very slowly down the drillpipe. (Once the drillpipe is clear of slurry, pump down both the drillpipe and the annulus.) If the rig pumps are used for the

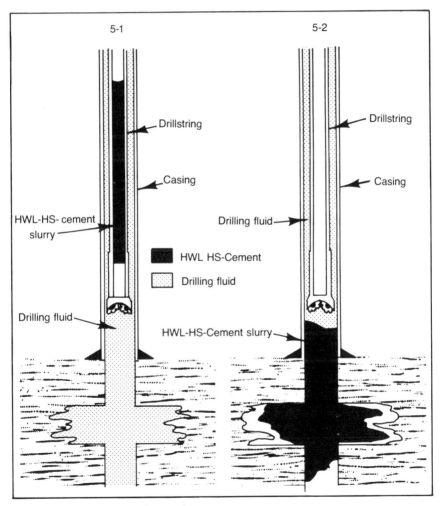

Fig. 5–1   HWL-HS-cement slurry at bit.
Fig. 5–2   HWL-HS-cement squeezed into formation.

squeeze, a mud gun should be left open to control surges. Attach a 0–500 psi pressure gauge to the annulus so that low pressures can be read accurately. If it is certain that all of the slurry is below the drillpipe, hold the squeeze for 30–60 min, pull clear, and WOC for 4–8 hours.

10) Pull out of the hole, pick up a bit, and go back to drilling. If there is no evidence of improvement after two batches, proceed to techniques 4, 6, 7C, or 7D (4, 5, 6, or 7 if water-base mud has been used.)

Technique 3B—High-Filter-Loss, Oil-Base Spacer Squeeze

Be assured, there's no such material. But that should not keep an operator from reaching for the most he can get. I have had his experience with Invermul (Baroid's inverted mud) and EZ-Spot (Baroid's oil-phase spacer). The HTHP API filter loss of Invermul at formation temperature was about 1 cc, while that of EZ-Spot, which contains no Invermul, was about 30 cc. This is not a great difference. But where the operator is building mud volume, there seems to be no reason for not taking advantage of this. It's cheaper too! While it has not been investigated in detail, this should apply to the oil-phase spacers of other mud suppliers as well. Look for an extension of the use of this property of oil-base spacers in Chapter 6.

Technique 4—Cements (Neat, Extended, Thixotropic, and Mix Your Own)

Use this technique against complete losses and severe complete losses to horizontal and some vertical loss zones. All cement slurries applied must be pumpable and have at least a safe minimum thickening time. There are no exceptions. The composition and technique of application of the cement slurry being used to combat lost circulation must be functionally adequate if the job is to succeed.

Cement Slurry Composition

Cement, neat alone and neat plus bentonite, is an important lost-circulation material because there are zones that it will effectively cure; both cement and bentonite are readily available at every well site. Because these two materials are relatively cheap and are universally available, they can be extremely useful in combating lost circulation, particularly if they are applied correctly.

There are many different additives for portland cement slurries— to make them lighter or heavier, to retard or accelerate their set, to lower their filter loss, to induce bridging properties into them, and to increase or decrease their gel strength. There are other kinds of cements such as organic polymers and gypsum. Any of these latter cements and any portland-plus additive mixture can be used to combat mud loss if they are available and are functionally suitable for the type of loss encountered.

Four portland cement slurries are recommended: neat, extended, thixotropic, and mix your own. These have been chosen because a wide variety of properties can be obtained by using them, and they usually are available.

Technique 4—Neat-Portland Cement

Mix to 15.6–15.8 lb/gal 46 to 44 wt % water based on cement. This slurry is dense, fluid, and develops high compressive strength when it sets.

Technique 4A—Extended Cements

BENTONITE OR ATTAPULGITE CEMENT

Bentonite cement formed by adding cement to water containing prehydrated bentonite gives optimum properties. The slurry has lower density, higher gel strength, and higher set strength than a slurry formed by adding water to a dry mixture of bentonite and cement.

In mixing the slurry, if required, treat the fresh water to be used with ¼ lb/bbl sodium carbonite and ¼ lb/bbl caustic to remove calcium and magnesium ions. Add 10 lb/bbl of bentonite and allow it to yield. Use this bentonite slurry to mix a 14.5 to 15.0 lb/gal bentonite-cement slurry. Use 100 sacks of cement or more for large hole sizes.

Attapulgite salt clay can be used as a substitute for bentonite in fresh or sea water. It is not flocculated by calcium ion so it gives the same yield whether it is added to the mix water or to the dry cement. Preshearing and prehydrating bentonite in fresh water and preshearing and preaging attapulgite in fresh or sea water (or brines) will markedly improve their yields and the properties of the cement slurries prepared from them.

PORTLAND CEMENT WITH AGGREGATES

Gilsonite or ground coal. Gilsonite or ground coal (Dowell's Kolite) can be added to cement slurries that are being used to regain returns. They decrease the density of the slurry and act as bridging agents; both of these functions help keep the slurry in the vicinity of the well bore. They should be run exactly like bentonite cement slurries and should be squeezed if the hole fills during application.

The composition and properties of gilsonite-portland cement admixtures are shown in Table 5–2. Between 25–100 lb of gilsonite per sack of cement are recommended.

TABLE 5–2 Composition and Properties of Gilsonite-Portland Cement Admixtures

Gilsonite (lb/sack of cement)	Water content of slurry (vol %)	Mixing water (wt %)*	Mixing water (gal/sack of cement)	Slurry volume (cu ft/sack of cement)	Slurry density (lb/gal)	Compressive strength (psi) in 24 hr at 100° F.
0	59.2	46.1	5.20	1.18	15.6	2,570
50	43.2	61.8	7.00	2.17	12.5	1,165
100	37.8	79.7	9.00	3.18	11.5	605
200	33.3	115	13.00	5.22	10.3	290

*Based on weight of dry cement

These four cements are recommended because they provide slurries with a range of properties from thin, heavy slurries which set hard to lighter, thick slurries having bridging properties. They are also available in many areas. But it is not intended that they be used to the exclusion of all other cement formulations.

One note about gilsonite and ground coal: it is safer to spot slurries containing these additives through open-end drillpipe. Amounts greater than 10 lb/94-lb sack can plug bits and float equipment.

TABLE 5–3 Slurry Properties of Cementing Composition for Normal Well Applications

Test slurry				Calculated slurry density (ppg) 2,000 psi	80°F, 24-hr compressive strength, psi
Spherelite, lb	Cement	Water (gal)	Other		
80	94 lb Class H	25.5*	4% CaCl$_2$	9.5	50
50	94 lb Class H	21.3**	3.5% CaCl$_2$	10.00	75
80	95 lb Class H	12.2	3% CaCl$_2$	10.00	151
60	95 lb Class H	10.3	3% CaCl$_2$	10.63	172
45	94 lb Class H	8.8	3% CaCl$_2$	11.23	254
35	94 lb Class H	7.9	3% CaCl$_2$	11.61	390
60	90 lb Fondu™	10.3	- - -	10.45	631
45	90 lb Fondu	8.8	- - -	11.03	727
35	90 lb Fondu	7.9	- - -	11.40	800

* Plus 6% Econolite additive, w/c = 0.4C + 2.18 Spherelite, no CFR-2 additive.
** Plus 4% Econolite, w/c = 0.4C + 2.80 Spherelite, no CFR-2 additive.
80°F compressive strengths of lightweight slurries prepared with Spherelite cement
All slurries mixed at w/c = 0.40 cement + 0.80 Spherelite. All samples cured at 80°F at 2,000 psi. All slurries contained 0.4% CFR-2 friction reducer based on the weight of cement (after Halliburton)

Frac sand. Frac sand is a material usually available in the field. Added to cement slurries in the amount of 10–20 lb/94-lb sack, 10–20-mesh frac sand will many times provide the bridging property required to start the bridge against which dehydration starts, with the result that the fracture is then packed with dry solids.

Hollow spheres. Halliburton offers the industry hollow inorganic spheres under the tradename Spherelite. The following advantages are claimed for it:

1) Compatible with all API cements and cement additives
2) Improved early compressive strength
3) Allows superlightweight slurries, 8–12 ppg
4) Will stand up to 6,000 psi
5) Insulates against heat and has application at ultrahigh temperatures
6) Is a lost circulation aid
7) Acts as an extender (bulk density is 25 lb/cu ft)

The slurry properties of Spherelite cementing compositons for normal well applications are shown in Table 5–3.

Technique 4B—Thixotropic Cements

Thixotropic cement slurries flow easily when being pumped and gel when pumping is stopped. This thixotropy gives several beneficial results when these cements are being applied to cure a loss zone. First, tha annular column of cement raised past a loss zone gels and does not fall back into the loss zone. Second, these cements have a greater tendency to pry induced vertical fractures apart and remain proximate to the well bore when applied against horizontal loss zones.

A typical composition of a thixotropic cement is

1) 90 parts Class A cement with a C_3A content of at least 5%
2) 10 parts gypsum
3) 1–3 parts calcium chloride

Overall, thixotropic cements are more effective against vertical and horizontal loss zones than the conventional portland cements. Why, then, are they not my first choice? There are two reasons: 1) They are not widely available at this writing, and 2) they have a depth limitation because retarders destroy their thixotropy. B.J. Hughes' Thixofil can be retarded.

Technique 4C—Mix Your Own Cement

Table 5–4 shows a fairly complete list of cement additives. The reader is invited to mix his own cement provided that it is pumpable and has a safe minimum thickening time.

TABLE 5–4   Cement Additives

Cement accelerators
Purpose: Reduce waiting on cement
       Increase early strength
1. Calcium chloride
2. Sodium chloride
3. Sodium silicate
4. Ammonium chloride
5. Gypsum cement
Cement retarders
Purpose: Increase thickening time
       Retard setting
1. Calcium lignosulfonates
2. Modified lignins
3. CMHEC (carboxymethyl-hydroxethyl
   cellulose)
4. Saturated salt water
5. Organic acid
Turbulence inducers or dispersants
1. Alkyl aryl sulfonates
2. Polyphosphates
3. Lignosulfonate
4. Lactones and gluconates
5. Synthetic polymers
6. Organic acids
Lightweight additives
Purpose: Reduce slurry weight
       Increase yield
       Lower costs
1. Attapulgite-bentonite
2. Pozzolans
3. Gilsonite
4. Expanded perlite
5. Diatomaceous earth
6. Hydrocarbons (emulsions)
7. Trinity Lite-Wate
8. Hollow Spheres
Heavyweight additives
Purpose: Increase density
       Restrain pressure

1. Hematite
2. Barite
3. Sand (40–60 mesh)
4. Saturated salt water
Filter loss additives
Purpose: Protect sensitive formations
       Prevent premature dehydration
       Better squeeze jobs
1. CMHEC (carboxymethyl-hydroxethyl
   cellulose)
2. Latex
3. Acrylic type copolymers
4. Organic polymer blends
Lost circulation additives
Purpose: Restore circulation
       Increased fill-up in column
       Reduce costs
1. Gilsonite
2. Granulated nut hulls
3. Cellophane flakes
4. Expanded perlites
5. Shredded fibers
6. Bentonite
7. Bentonite diesel oil
8. Hollow spheres
Special additives
1. Radioactive tracers
2. Activated charcoal
3. Paraformaldehyde—sodium
   chromate
4. Silica flour
Special cements
1. Gypsum cement
2. Resin cement
3. Diesel-oil cement
4. Pozzolan-lime cements (for high
   temperatures)
5. Densified

Techniques for Applying Cement

Cement slurries should be used to combat losses to natural horizontal fractures ⅓ in. to 1 ft in diameter and to broken limestones or to boulders.

Cementing loss zones results in failure many times because mud has broken through the unset slurry. Balancing columns and dropping the plug will usually prevent this, particularly if column weights are carefully calculated.

BALANCED-COLUMN METHOD

1. If possible, drill without returns through all the lost-circulation zone.

2. Pull out of the hole. Measure the static mud level using a piece of wood (4 in. by 4 in. by 4 ft) on a wire line. Put on a cementing sub consisting of 2 ft of appropriate size drillpipe with a cap welded over its lower end and perforated with four 1-in. wide by 3-in. high windows just above the cap in the sides of the drillpipe.

3. Choose a cement slurry. According to the severity of the loss zone, mix and run 100–300 sacks.

4. Locate the loss zone. (a) By temperature survey: Wait 4 hours, and then run the temperature profile of the open hole. Pump in 100 bbl of mud through the fill-up line and rerun the profile. The loss is occurring at the temperature discontinuity.

(b) By gamma-ray log and radioactive material: If the loss zone is suspected to be near the top of the hole, pump 15 bbl of mud containing radioactive material down the annulus; use the log inside the drillpipe to follow the progress of the material downhole. If you suspect the zone is at the bottom of the hole, pump the radioactive slug down the drillpipe.

After the slug has been displaced out of the drillpipe, lower the gamma-ray log and follow the progress of the material up the annulus. It may be necessary to pump down both the annulus and drillpipe before the loss zone can be located. The drillpipe should be reciprocated during logging and pumping to prevent it from sticking.

5. Run the drillpipe and cementing sub past the loss zone to make sure it's exposed. Clean the hole past the zone if required. As shown in Fig. 5–3, set the cementing sub at a point 50 ft above the top of the loss zone.

6. Mix just enough cement slurry to hydrostatically balance the mud column in the annulus. Wait 5 min with pumps shut down while cement falls to the end of the drillpipe and the pumping mud level falls to the static mud level (Fig. 5–4). At this point, the mud and cement column in the drillpipe just balances the mud column in the annulus.

Mix the remainder of the cement and displace at 10 bbl/min with enough mud so that 2 bbl of cement (140 ft for 4½-in. pipe) are left in the drillpipe (there is always the possibility that some or all the cement will come up around the drillpipe). The cement left in the drillpipe will fill the void the pipe leaves as it is withdrawn. Otherwise, the void will fill with mud. This would weaken the cement by forming a channel through it to the loss zone).

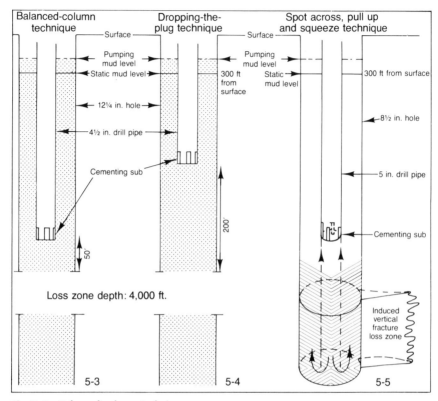

Fig. 5–3 **Balanced-column technique**
Fig. 5–4 **Dropping-the-plug technique**
Fig. 5–5 **Spot-across, pull-up, and squeeze technique**

If the amount of cement mixed is not sufficient to balance the mud column in the annulus, the cement slurry must be displaced to the point where the displacement mud plus the cement does. Then, after waiting 5 min, finish displacing with mud at 10 bbl/min without interruption or breaking any lines. Leave 2 bbl of cement in the drillpipe.

7. Pull out of the hole. As the pipe is withdrawn, the mud level in the annulus will fall and cause an imbalance of pressure from the formation to the hole, which may cause mud or formation fluids to break through the cement slurry. To prevent this, very carefully add mud to the annulus through the fill-up line.

Adding too much mud to the annulus will force mud from the annulus into the formation through the cement slurry before it has a chance to set. The amount of mud pumped must match the volume displacement (not capacity) of the pipe. If it is done carelessly, it can do more harm than good. Pump the required amount of mud every 10 stands. Wait on cement at least 8 hours.

8. Measure fluid level. If it is lower or higher than the original static level, do not attempt to adjust. If it is higher and another plug is run, adjust by adding proportionately less mud as the pipe is withdrawn.

DROPPING-THE-PLUG TECHNIQUE

Dropping the plug depends on the excess weight of the cement column over that of the mud it displaces. The cement plug falls down the hole into the loss zone when pumping is stopped and balances with approximately ⅙ to ⅓ of the cement in the hole and ⅚ to ⅔ of the cement in the formation.

This technique should not be used, particularly in large-diameter holes (12¼-in. and up), if the mud weight is over 11 lb/gal or with small amounts of cement (100 sacks or less).

This technique is similar to the balanced-column technique. Here's how it should be run:

1. If possible, drill without returns through all the lost-circulation zone.

2. Pull out of the hole. Measure the static mud level using a piece of wood (4 in. by 4 in. by 4 ft) on a wire line. Put on a cementing sub consisting of 2 ft of appropriate-sized drillpipe with a cap welded over its lower end and perforated with four 1-in.-wide by 3-in.-high windows just above the cap in the sides of the drillpipe.

3. Choose a cement slurry. According to the severity of the loss zone, mix and run 100–300 sacks.

4. Locate the loss zone as in Step 4, balanced-column method.

5. Run the drillpipe and cementing sub past the loss zone to make sure it is exposed. Clean the hole past the zone if required. As shown in Fig. 5–4, set the cementing sub at a point 200 ft above the top of the loss zone.

6. Mix just enough cement slurry to hydrostatically balance the mud column in the annulus. Wait 5 min with pumps shut down while cement falls to the end of the drillpipe and the mud level in the annulus falls from the pumping level to the static pressure level.

Mix the remainder of the cement and displace at 10 bbl/min with enough mud so that 2 bbl of cement (140 ft for 4½-in. pipe) are left in the drillpipe and the mud and cement column in the drillpipe just balances the mud column in the annulus. If the amount of cement mixed is not sufficient to balance the mud column in the annulus, the cement slurry must be displaced to the point where the displacement mud plus the cement provides this balance. Then after waiting 5 min, finish displacing the mud at 10 bbl/min without interruption or breaking any lines. Leave 2 bbl of cement in the drillpipe.

It is very important when using this technique to displace, after the 5-min rest period, at a fast rate (10 bbl/min) without interruption and without beaking any lines. The cement plug adds weight to the static mud column and depends on pumping pressure to remain in equilibrium. If pumping is interrupted, the mud in the annulus will fall past the cementing sub; when pumping is resumed there will be a spot of mud in the cement column.

7. Pull out of the hole. As the pipe is withdrawn, the mud level in the annulus will fall and cause an imbalance of pressure from the formation to the hole that may cause mud or formation fluids to break through the cement slurry. To prevent this, very carefully add mud to the annulus through the fill-up line.

Adding too much mud to the annulus will force mud from the annulus into the formation through the cement slurry before the cement has a chance to set. The amount of mud pumped must match the volume displacement (not capacity) of the pipe. If it is done carelessly, it can do more harm than good. Pump the required amount of mud every 10 stands. Wait on the cement at least 8 hours.

8. Measure fluid level. If it is lower or higher than the original static level, do not attempt to adjust. If it is higher and another plug is run, adjust by adding proportionately less mud as the pipe is withdrawn.

It is not possible to foresee every possibility or describe all cements in these instructions. Success will always depend on those engineering the job to be alert to significant factors that develop during the job and that are peculiar to the job. Cement should be used only where the loss zone is severe enough for the cement slurry to enter under its own weight. Accordingly, mud returns during the job should not be expected.

If returns are obtained during a job, the cement should be displaced and the pipe raised to a point near the top of the cement plug. Care should be taken not to leave a core of mud in the cement slug. The rams should be closed and the cement carefully squeezed into the loss zone.

Where no cement will stay in the hole, either of techniques 3, 5, 6, or 7 can be followed by technique 4. Soft plugs such as diesel oil-bentonite slurry are used as backing material to hold the cement round the well bore.

At the completion of the application of any lost-circulation materials, the drillpipe is essentially full of drilling mud. Subsequent materials will force this mud through lost-circulation materials already in place and impair earlier jobs.

Accordingly, the best possible way to follow techniques 3, 5, 6, or 7 with technique 4 (cement) is to run the cement slurry immediately following, that is, without displacing the other material.

If the risk of the cement setting in the drillpipe is too great, the first plug must be displaced. But then to get the cement into the loss zone the volume of mud the drillpipe holds must be pumped through the plug just displaced.

Calculations required for balancing columns

To be able to balance one column of liquids with another, the height and density of each must be known. In the drillpipe, the amount of cement and mud in the column and the densities of each are known.

In the annulus, however, accurate calculations depend on finding the static level of the mud below the flow nipple. Once this is established, the average density of the mud in the annulus must be estimated. This is difficult only if this mud has been gas-cut or partially displaced with a lighter or heavier mud after circulation was lost.

Sample calculations are given below in terms of a typical loss zone. Note that the calculations are dependent on the hole size, static mud level, mud density, cement slurry density, amount of cement, amount of mud used for displacement, and the depth of the loss zone.

The static mud level and density of the mud are very important, and an effort should be made to determine them accurately.

1. Physical conditions existing:

Drillpipe (DP) size, in. (16.60 lb)	4½ (cap. in ft/bbl = 70)
Hole size, in.	12¼ (cap. in ft/bbl = 6.86)
Mud density, lb/gal	9.0 (46.8 psi/100 ft)
Cement slurry density, lb/gal	14.5 (75.5 psi/100 ft)
Static fluid level, ft	300
Depth of lost-circulation zone, ft	4,000
DP displacement, gal/joint	7.65
Sacks of cement	260
Volume of bentonite slurry used, bbl	34
Volume of cement slurry, bbl	260/10 + 34 = 60
Feet of open hole cement slurry will fill	411
Feet of drillpipe cement slurry will fill	4,200

2. Barrels of cement slurry in drillpipe needed to just balance mud column in the annulus (end of drillpipe 50 ft above top of loss zone):

Feet of mud column: 3,650

Weight of mud column, psi:

$$3,650 \times 0.052 \times 9.0 = 1,710$$

$$1,710 \text{ psi} = \text{feet of cement slurry} \times 0.052 \times 14.5$$

$$\text{Feet of slurry} = \frac{1,710}{14.5 \times 0.052}$$

$$\text{Barrels of slurry} = \frac{1,710}{14.5 \times 0.052 \times 70} = 32.4$$

3. Remainder of cement slurry: $60 - 32.4 = 27.6$ bbl.

4. Barrels of mud required to displace all but 2 bbl of the cement slurry.

$$1,710 \text{ psi} = \text{feet of mud in DP} \times 9.0 \times 0.052 + \text{ft of cement slurry}$$
$$(140) \text{ in DP} \times 0.052 \times 14.5$$

Feet of mud in DP =

$$\frac{1,710 - (0.052 \times 14.5) \,(140)}{9.0 \times 0.052}$$

$$= \frac{1,605}{9.0 \times 0.052} = 3,440$$

$$\text{Barrels of displacement mud} = \frac{3,440}{70} = 49 \text{ bbl}$$

Capacity of 3,950 ft of 4½-in. DP = 56.5 bbl.

5. Drillpipe displacement: Displacement of 16.60-lb 4½-in. drillpipe is 7.65 gal/30 ft including upsets and couplings:

$$\text{DP displacement} = \frac{3,650}{30} \times \frac{7.65}{42}$$

$$= 22 \text{ bbl}$$

Pump 5½ bbl of mud every 10 stands while coming out of the hole.

6. Cement level drop: When the dropping-the-plug technique is used just after displacement, the following conditions apply:

Length of the mud column in the annulus is 3,500 ft.

Length of the cement slurry column below DP is 200 ft.

Weight of the mud column to the top of the loss zone, psi:

$$(3,700 \times 0.052 \times 9.0) = 1,730.$$

Weight of mud and cement column, psi = $(3,500 \times 9.0 + 200 \times 14.5)$ $0.052 = (31,500 + 2,900) \, 0.052 = (34,400) \, 0.052 = 1,790$

Cement-level drop $= \dfrac{(1,790 - 1,730)}{0.052 \times 14.5} = 80$ ft

Cement remaining in the hole = 120 ft or

$\dfrac{120}{6.86} = 17.5$ bbl

Cement in loss zone = $60 - 17.5 = 42.5$ bbl

Spot Across, Pull Up, and Squeeze Technique

On occasion, cement slurries are also effective in combating mud losses to induced vertical fractures, particularly if the fractured zone is porous. If it is not, possibly an aggregate should be added to the cement slurry. Earlier, it was demonstrated that to seal an induced vertical fracture and improve its integrity, the fracture must be pried apart and held apart either while the loss agent dehydrates or sets. This can be accomplished by spotting the cement slurry across the loss zone, pulling up, and then applying a hesitation squeeze (Fig. 5–5). If the hole has filled during the spotting of the cement slurry, the BOP's can then be closed and the hesitation squeeze applied. A sought for squeeze pressure high enough to proceed with the drilling operation should be fixed; when it is attained, it should be held while WOC. Pump ¼-bbl increments with 15-min waits in between. Retard the slurry if required for squeeze time. If it is easy to squeeze the cement slurry away, use a high-filter-loss slurry; if it is difficult, use a low-filter-loss slurry.

Case History

In the subject well offshore North Africa, 9⅝-inch casing was set at 13,385 feet and an 8½-inch hole was drilled to 14,254 feet. Five hesitation squeezes had repaired loss zones in the upper hole, but due to a bridge a loss zone still existed near the bottom of the hole. A 16.5-lb/gal inverted emulsion mud was in use; loss zones were to induced vertical fractures in sand, shale, and dolomite. A stinger (704 feet) of 2⅞-inch tubing with a mill end was run to 14,225 feet and 55 bbl of cement slurry mixed. Of this, 47 bbl were displaced up around the tubing and 8 bbl were left in it.

The mill was pulled then to a point above the top of the slurry and the tubing cleared. Next, the mill was pulled into the casing. From this vantage point, 11 bbl of cement slurry (5 on annulus, 6 on drillpipe) were squeezed into the formations. An annular pressure of 250 psi developed, which was held while WOC. The plug was drilled out, full circulation was restored, and a leak-off test showed the hole would now hold a 17.5 mud equivalent. To prevent imbalances between the drillpipe and the annulus, the mud, the spacer, and the cement were designed and mixed to weigh the same 16.5 lb/gal.

Technique 5—Downhole-Mixed Soft-Hard Plugs (M+DOB2C)[15,16]

Techniques 5 and 5A can be used against complete losses and severe complete losses to horizontal and vertical loss zones. M+DOB2C is widely used; M+DOAB4C has limited application. Accordingly in the discussion that follows, reference is almost wholly to M+DOB2C.

In the formula M+DOB2C (1:2), the M refers to the mud component.* It can be fresh or sea water or any water-base drilling mud, whatever its weight or composition. The M component varies from job to job. The DOB2C component consists of one 100-lb sack of bentonite and two 94-lb sacks of portland cement mixed in 26.5 gal of diesel oil to form a slurry weighing 12.4 lb/gal.

Density and Yield Calculations

The density and yield calculations for DOB2C are shown in Table 5–5:

Table 5–5   Density and Yield Calculations for DOB2C

Volume of material, gal	Specific volume, gal/lb	Weight of material, lb	Material	Diesel oil requirement, gal
4.53	0.0453	100	Wyoming bentonite	26.5
7.18	0.0382	188	Class G cement	
		185.5	Diesel oil	11.71
11.71		473.5		38.21

Slurry density, lb/gal, equals 12.4
Slurry yield, cu ft/100-lb sack bentonite, equals 5.11
Bbl of slurry/bbl of diesel oil equals 1.44

*The 1:2 component of M+DOB2C (1:2) is the ratio of mud (M) to DOB2C.

56

Pilot Testing M+DOB2Cs

Prior to applying M+DOB2C to a well, pilot tests of various mud to DOB2C ratios are run using the mud and DOB2C on location. For example, the following ratios would be tested by measuring the mud and DOB2C into a mud cup in the correct proportions and then stirring and kneading the mixture until all the diesel oil breaks out. Typical results for fresh water and DOB2C would be for mud: DOB2C:

       1:1 ---------- soft
       1:1½---------- medium
       1:2 ---------- medium to hard
       1:2½---------- hard
       1:3 ---------- very hard

(Use separate cups for measuring the mud and DOB2C.)

From these tests an M+DOB2C (1:X) soft enough to seek the loss zone yet hard enough to seal it is chosen. Also chosen is an M+DOB2C (1:X) hard enough to plug the open hole. In Plates 1–7, a series of M+DOB2Cs ranging from soft to very hard is shown to help one

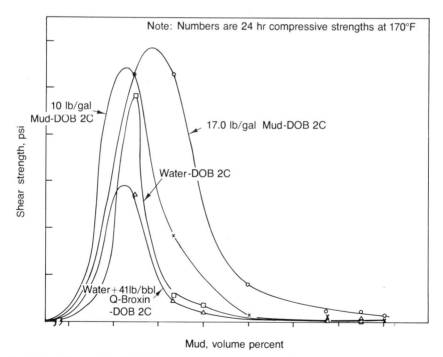

Fig. 5–6 Effect of M+DOB2C ratio on shear strength of hand-mixed mixture. DOB2C weighed 12.3 ppg and contained a ratio of two 94-lb sacks of class A cement to one 100-lb sack of bentonite

choose the right ratios. The shear strength data in Fig. 5–6 of hand-mixed Mud-DOB2Cs will be of further help.

Obviously, the reason 26.5 gal of diesel oil are used in the slurry is that it makes a pumpable slurry in which the solids are satisfactorily suspended. But why the ratio of 1 100-lb sack of Wyoming bentonite to 2 94-lb sacks of cement when DOBC and DOB3C were used earlier?

Bentonite to Cement Ratio

Be aware that there are an infinite number of ratios of bentonite to cement as we go from diesel oil-cement (DOC) to diesel oil-bentonite (DOB) (Fig. 5–7). Actually, we are seeking an M+DOB(X)C that will form a highly gelled mass when it is mixed with mud that will pry the fracture apart and then set and develop compressive strength to hold it apart. The bentonite gives the pry (the gel strength) and the cement the set (the compressive strength). Based on its very satisfactory performance in the field, M+DOB2C appears to have near-optimum properties of both of these. Thus, the ratio of bentonite to cement in DOB2C is not the optimum, but mixed in the correct proportion with any water-base mud it works.

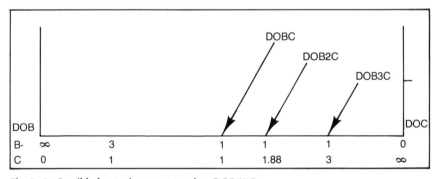

Fig. 5–7 Possible bentonite-cement ratios, DOB(X)Cs

Reasons for M+DOB2C Failures

As stated earlier, if M+DOB2C can be squeezed into an induced vertical fracture at a positive pressure so as to pry the fracture apart and hold the sought-for squeeze pressure until the M+DOB2C sets, it has always (in my experience) sealed the loss zone. However, there have been many instances of reported failures when the sought-for squeeze pressures have been developed. Usually this is because the M+DOB2C (1:X) was too hard and plugged the open hole before it reached the loss zone (Fig. 5–8). To avoid this, M+DOB2C (1:X) should first be mixed soft enough to seek, yet hard enough to seal the loss zone before it is

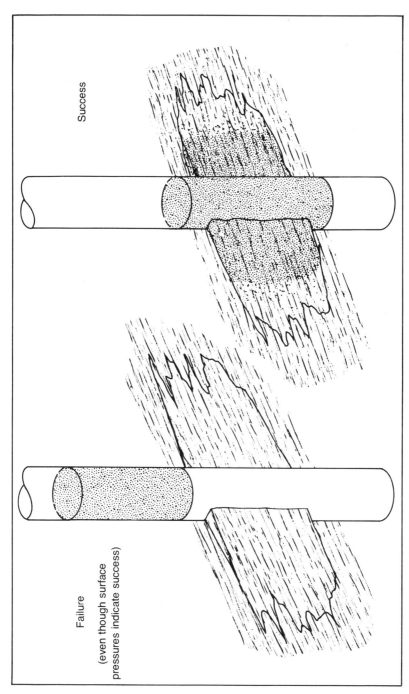

Fig. 5–8   M+DOB2C too thick (left), plugging the open hole. (Right) M+DOB2C thin enough to seek and enter, thick enough to seal.

mixed hard enough to plug the open hole. Of course, another reason for failure is that all the loss zone was not available because of a bridge in the hole.

DOB2C Additives

For most applications, DOB2C is best to use. However, there are instances where it would be advantageous to (a) densify the DOB2C and still have it pumpable to deliver more active solids to the problem, (b) have better suspension of its solids where premixed DOB2C needs to be stored, (c) lower its filter loss to avoid dehydration at leaks in the string or at restrictions as in a core barrel, (d) have it less active to slight amounts of water where the diesel oil is wet as it was in Sumatra, and (e) react more slowly when mixed with mud to give the M+DOB2C formed from it greater reach down hole. All these properties can be achieved by adding any of the oil-base dispersants shown in Table 5–6 and/or an oleophilic bentonite such as Baroid's Geltone to the DOB2C. Since the need for these additives is limited, detailed information for achieving the above results are not given in the text. Rather, the reader is referred to Reference 15, in which the effects of these materials on DOB2C, DOB and DOC are presented in detail.

TABLE 5–6   Dispersant Description*

Tradename of dispersant	Distributor	Chemical composition	Density, lb/gal cost	Estimated amount required in plug, lb/final bbl
EZ-Mul	Baroid	Half amide salt terminated	8.1 0.455	0.5
Driltreat	Bariod	Lecithin	8.7 0.572	0.5
Surf-Cote	Milchem	Oil-soluble amine dodecyl benzene sulfonate	8.16 1.22	1.0
SA-47	Oil Base, Inc.	Aryl alkyl sodium sulfonate**	8.12 0.88	0.5
Fazethin	Magcobar			1.0
Ken-Thin	Imco	Imidazolin	7.9 0.925	1.5
SE-11	Magcobar	Modified alkyl aryl sulfonate plus imidazolin	7.83 0.93	1.5
Carbo-Mul	Milchem	Oil-soluble alkanol amide	7.5 0.601	1.5

*Listed in the order of effectiveness; however, all are recommended for use.
**U.S. Patent No. 3,099,624

Methods of Mixing DOB2C

DOB2C is formulated by mixing 1 100-lb sack of bentonite, 2 94-lb sacks of cement, and 26.5 gal of diesel oil together to form a 12.4 lb/gal slurry. This can be done in 3 ways: (a) batch mixing, (b) making a dry blend of the bentonite and the cement (B2C) and hopper mixing it with the diesel oil, or (c) adding the bentonite to the diesel oil to form a DOB of the correct composition and then adding the cement to it across a hopper.

Batch mixing. When DOB2C is batch mixed, it is usually in the cementer's tanks. Proceed as follows:

1) Place 13.86 bbl diesel oil in the tanks
2) Add 21.96 100-lb sacks of bentonite
3) Add 43.92 94-lb sacks of cement

This yields 20 bbl of 12.4 lb/gal DOB2C. Of course larger amounts can be batch mixed if desired.

Hopper-mix B2C into diesel oil. Prepare a B2C blend in a cement bin; add it to diesel oil coming across the hopper to form a 12.4 lb/gal DOB2C slurry continuously.

Hopper-mix cement into a DOB. Form a DOB by adding bentonite to diesel oil in the ratio of 100 lb of bentonite to 26.5 gal of diesel oil. To mix 100 bbl of 12.4-ppg DOB2C, mix 81.13 bbl of DOB (don't forget to scale up for what is not deliverable) in a 150-bbl tank as follows:

1) Place 69.28 bbl of diesel oil into the tank
2) Add 109.8 100-lb sacks of bentonite
3) Hopper mix 219.6 94-lb sacks of cement into the DOB to form 100 bbls of 12.4-ppg DOB2C.

Of the three methods of mixing DOB2C, hopper mixing B2C blend into diesel oil is the least frought with problems. Assuming there is an adequate supply of diesel oil to the cementing unit, the truck is flushed free of water and mud, the tanks are filled with 20 bbl of diesel oil, the 10 bbl of diesel oil ahead is pumped into the drillpipe, and the tank is refilled. Now the required amount of DOB2C is hopper mixed continuously into the drillpipe and 5 bbl of diesel oil are pumped behind. The cementer's tanks are then filled with mud for displacing the DOB2C. There are several advantages. No water-reactive DOB2C or DOB gets out into the mud system where it can be gelled by water or mud leaking into it. Forming M+DOB2C or M+DOB in the mud lines is a situation to be avoided.

What about batch mixing DOB2C in the cementer's tanks? Provided that 20 bbl is enough, there still is a problem of measuring the diesel oil ahead and behind. One advantage that hopper mixing cement into DOB has is that any excess DOB can be used, in most circumstances, to make drilling mud. Excess B2C and particularly excess batch-mixed DOB2C must be discarded.

In the example M+DOB2C job described later, hopper mixing B2C into diesel oil continuously will be suggested. However, the other two methods can be used if they suit better and are more convenient.

Weighting DOB2C

Weighting materials such as barite can be used to increase the weight of DOB2C. Yet I have never run any weighted DOB2C. Rather, the mud in use, which can vary in weight from fresh water (8.33 ppg) to weighted drilling muds (up to 18.5 lb/gal), was just mixed with DOB2C to form M+DOB2Cs of the correct consistency.

Having the DOB2C lighter than the drilling mud in use is an advantage when applying DOB2C. If the mud column in the annulus is heavier than the mud-diesel oil-DOB2C column in the drillpipe, the DOB2C remains stationary if pumping is interrupted. When the drilling mud is lighter (sea water, for example), the DOB2C continues to fall if pumping is stopped, making it more difficult to know just when and at what rate the DOB2C reaches the mixing point. Thus, it is more difficult to pump the correct amount of mud to it down the annulus.

DOB2C-carrying Bridging Agents

Of course bridging agents can be added to DOB2C. However, M+DOB2C will plug more severe loss zones than can be plugged by bridging agents in mud (technique 2) or high-filter-loss slurry squeeze (technique 3). Carried by a highly gelled M+DOB2C, it is doubtful if bridging agents would be more apt to form a bridge than when applied in mud or high-filter-loss slurry. This probably would weaken rather than improve the compressive strength of set M+DOB2C. Further, they could prevent, by filtering out on the faces, the M+DOB2C from entering smaller fractures and prying them apart as the squeeze pressure increases. The reader may use them if he wants; but I have never added bridging agents to the M+DOB2Cs I apply.

Adequate Supply of Diesel Oil

Would you undertake a cement job with mixing and displacing equipment-supplied displacement mud and mix water through a 1-inch line? Of course not. But this is usually the situation in regard to supplying diesel oil to the mud pits and the cementing unit when mixing DOB2C. To mix DOB2C in the right amount at the right rate, diesel oil must be supplied to the cementing unit and mud pits by at least a 3-inch line supplied by an adequate pump. Using B2C and diesel oil, a Halliburton unit can mix DOB2C at a rate of 7½ bbl/min. To do this continuously, it must be supplied diesel oil at a rate of 5.21 bbl/min. Insist on this; it will pay for the installation many times over.

Amount of M+DOB2C to Run

1) Minimum amount would be twice the volume of the open hole to be treated plus the volume to be left in the casing.

2) For complete losses—30–70 bbl of M+DOB2C

3) For severe complete losses—70–150 bbl of M+DOB2C

4) For very severe losses—150–300 bbl of M+DOB2C

In the final analysis, the amount of M+DOB2C run must be matched to the severity of the loss at the location. The amounts suggested above are guidelines only.

M+DOB2C Not Applicable where Oil Muds are in Use

Since a water-base mud (M) must be mixed with DOB2C to form M+DOB2C, the use of M+DOB2C to cure lost returns is not viable where oil muds are in use. Some say that a slug of water base mud can be spotted in the annulus above the loss zone prior to the bradenhead squeeze. But if the annulus is not full and there are severe losses, it is difficult—if not impossible—to control the ratio of water base mud to DOB2C.

Application of M+DOB2C

The steps below should be used when designing and applying a M+DOB2C squeeze. The presentation follows a question and answer format:

To successfully cure severe and very severe complete losses to natural horizontal and induced vertical fractures, one must apply the right amount of the right material at the right rate in the right place. Consider the following lost-circulation problem: 9⅝-in. casing had been set at 10,000 ft. One thousand feet of 8½-in. hole had been drilled below it when circulation was lost. A 10.0 lb/gal fresh-water mud was being used. Partial mud losses had occurred at 10,075 ft but had been sealed using bridging agents in mud (technique 2).

1) Make sure all of the lost circulation zone is exposed. Run in to bottom to be sure there is no fill. If it is the first time the loss zones have been encountered, if possible drill without returns through the loss zone.

2) Locate the loss zone; determine its type and severity. (It is a severe induced vertical fracture at about 10,075 ft.)

3) Choose the right lost-circulation material and technique (M+DOB2C, of course). Run the pilot tests using the 10.0 lb/gal mud and 12.4 ppg DOB2C. From these choose a lead slurry (M+DOB2C (1:1) is chosen) and a final slurry (M+DOB2C (1:2) is chosen) (Fig. 5–9).

4) Choose the amount of DOB2C (20 bbl). Prepare 300 96-lb sacks of B2C blend by adding 100 100-lb sacks of bentonite to 200 94-lb sacks

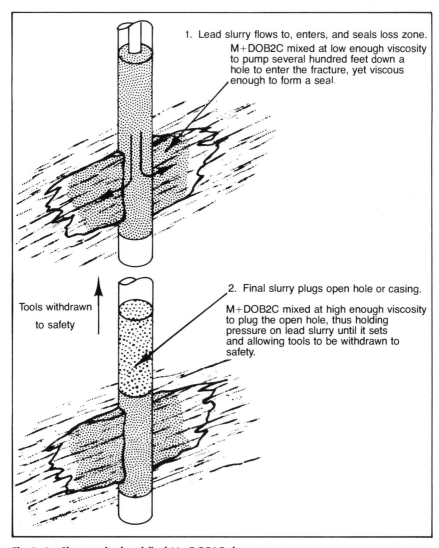

1. Lead slurry flows to, enters, and seals loss zone.

M+DOB2C mixed at low enough viscosity to pump several hundred feet down a hole to enter the fracture, yet viscous enough to form a seal.

Tools withdrawn to safety

2. Final slurry plugs open hole or casing.

M+DOB2C mixed at high enough viscosity to plug the open hole, thus holding pressure on lead slurry until it sets and allowing tools to be withdrawn to safety.

Fig. 5–9   Choose a lead and final M+DOB2C slurry.

of cement and blowing it back and forth between two bins. It could be dry-blended onshore and delivered to a bin on the rig. The DOB2C could be batch mixed or hopper mixed by adding cement to DOB if more convenient.

5) Pull out of the hole. Put on a mixing sub consisting of 5 ft of appropriate-sized drillpipe orange-peeled at the lower end and with four 1-in. by 4-in. slots cut 1 ft above the end (Fig. 5–10). DOB2C can be placed through a jet bit if required, but because of the complications of the drill collars, the danger of sticking the string is much greater.

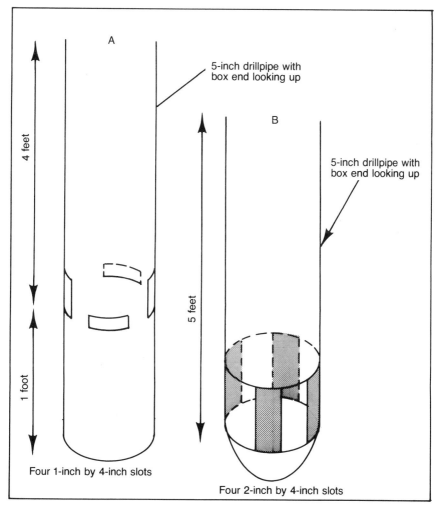

Fig. 5–10   M+DOB2C mixing sub designs

6) Set the bottom of the mixing sub 50–150 ft above the loss zone (9,925 ft that, in this example, is up in the 9⅝-in casing). Install a 0–2,000-psi gauge on the annulus.

7) Set a maximum squeeze pressure (1,500 psi).

8) Place 20 bbl of diesel oil in the cementer's tanks; pump 10 bbl of diesel oil ahead. Somewhat lesser amounts can be used at shallower depths but not less than 5 bbl. Refill the tank with diesel oil.

9) Using the B2C blend from the bin and diesel oil across the hopper, hopper mix 20 bbl of DOB2C into the drillpipe. Every barrel of diesel oil yields 1.44 bbl of 12.4-ppg DOB2C.

10) Pump 5 bbl of diesel oil behind the DOB2C.

11) Displace the slurry down the drillpipe at 10 bbl/min with *air-free* mud. Slow the rate to 3 bbl/min when the diesel oil reaches the mixing sub.

12) If there are no returns, simultaneously start pumping mud into the annulus at 3 bbl/min. Even if the hole fills and circulates (or if there are returns at the outset), continue pumping into the annulus at 3 bbl/min. When the diesel oil ahead reaches the mixing sub, close the rams. This is to avoid pumping 10 bbl of diesel oil, which will mix with the DOB2C instead of mud when the squeeze starts, up around the pipe.

Now start the squeeze procedure shown in Fig. 5–11. M+DOB2C correctly mixed and placed will plug an induced vertical fracture. However, it is difficult to judge how much mud is going past the mixing sub when pumping into the annulus when it is not full. One can be sure 3 bbl/min of mud are going past the mixing sub into the loss zone and the correct M+DOB2C can be formulated with the hole full, the rams closed and the mixing sub up in the casing. Another complication is that the column of mud, diesel oil, and DOB2C in the drillpipe can be heavier than the 10.0 ppg mud in the annulus. It may fall and reach the mixing sub before all the mud required to put the diesel oil at the mixing sub has been pumped.

Disposing of Excess DOB2C

I can recall only one instance where a troublesome amount of DOB2C could not be formed into M+DOB2C and pumped into the loss zone. In a well in Indonesia 54.5-lb K-40 13⅜-inch casing was set at 3,976 feet. Its internal yield was 2,730 psi. At the outset of the job, there were 600 psi on the BOPs and 16.7-ppg mud in use. Sixty bbl of DOBC were mixed into the drillpipe; at 30 bbl mixed with mud through the bit and pumped into the loss zone, a squeeze pressure of 2,400 psi

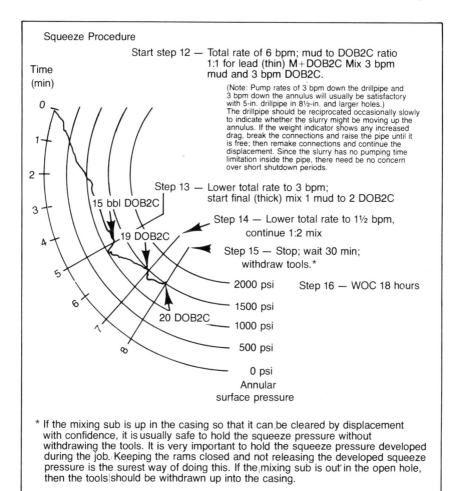

Squeeze Procedure

Time (min)

Start step 12 — Total rate of 6 bpm; mud to DOB2C ratio 1:1 for lead (thin) M+DOB2C Mix 3 bpm mud and 3 bpm DOB2C.

(Note: Pump rates of 3 bpm down the drillpipe and 3 bpm down the annulus will usually be satisfactory with 5-in. drillpipe in 8½-in. and larger holes.) The drillpipe should be reciprocated occasionally slowly to indicate whether the slurry might be moving up the annulus. If the weight indicator shows any increased drag, break the connections and raise the pipe until it is free; then remake connections and continue the displacement. Since the slurry has no pumping time limitation inside the pipe, there need be no concern over short shutdown periods.

15 bbl DOB2C

19 DOB2C

20 DOB2C

Step 13 — Lower total rate to 3 bpm; start final (thick) mix 1 mud to 2 DOB2C

Step 14 — Lower total rate to 1½ bpm, continue 1:2 mix

Step 15 — Stop; wait 30 min; withdraw tools.*

2000 psi   Step 16 — WOC 18 hours

1500 psi

1000 psi

500 psi

0 psi
Annular
surface pressure

* If the mixing sub is up in the casing so that it can be cleared by displacement with confidence, it is usually safe to hold the squeeze pressure without withdrawing the tools. It is very important to hold the squeeze pressure developed during the job. Keeping the rams closed and not releasing the developed squeeze pressure is the surest way of doing this. If the mixing sub is out in the open hole, then the tools should be withdrawn up into the casing.

Fig. 5–11   Squeeze procedure.

built up on the annulus and held. It was feared that higher pressures would rupture the casing, so the following was done to clear the drill-pipe:

Thirty bbl of 17.5-ppg mud were mixed and pumped into the drill-pipe; this killed the drillpipe as it forced the 30 bbl of DOBC out and up around the string. Simultaneously, 30 bbl of mud were bled from the annulus through the choke. Four stands of drillpipe were then stripped out through the BOPs while 15 bbl of mud were pumped into the annulus through the kill line. This forced the DOBC, which had reached

1,500 ft up around the string, below the bit. The string actually came free on the fourth stand, but it was necessary to pull 150,000 lb over the weight of the string.

Note: If a stand (90 ft) of wet 5-in. drillpipe is pulled through the BOPs, 2¼ bbl of mud must be pumped into the annulus through the kill line to replace this volume and force the gelled DOBC under the bit.

Fig. 5–12 shows how the mud the collars displace, when they are being pulled from the hole, must flow from above to below the collars while the collars are being withdrawn. If this does not occur, the well is being swabbed. In a clean hole with good mud, this occurs. But gelled DOBC above the collars will not flow by itself and must be forced. At the surface, if the drillpipe is pulling dry, the mud level in the annulus should fall 0.59 bbl/stand if the well is not being swabbed.

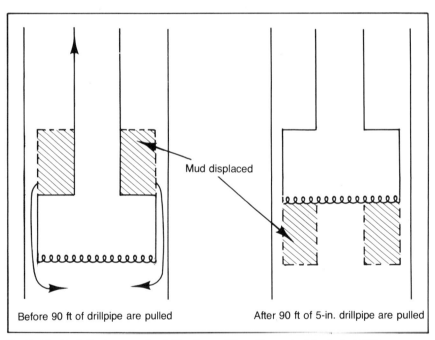

Before 90 ft of drillpipe are pulled   After 90 ft of 5-in. drillpipe are pulled

Fig. 5–12   Mud displacement by drill collars while pulling out of the hole (POH)

In summary, there are several possible means of disposing of excess DOB2C, DOAB2C, DOB, Bengum, and Polymer Plug. Rememb-ber that under most circumstances the ojbect would have been sealed. This allows one to operate safely above the plug.

68

1) Pull out of the hole, stringing the material in the drillpipe up the hole. This works whether the drillpipe is in open-ended with a mixing sub or with collars and a bit. Of course, the entire mud system is apt to be contaminated by this procedure.

2) Pump the material in the drillpipe up around the string and then pull out of the hole. This is practical if the drillpipe is in open-ended or with a mixing sub. However, if the drillpipe is in with collars and a bit, then to force the material under the bit as the drillpipe is withdrawn the string must be stripped out through the BOPs while mud is pumped into the annulus to replace the volume being withdrawn from the hole.

Case History

In the Gulf of Mexico lost returns to a series of depleted sands in an interval from 7,450–8,200 ft were cured using M (sea water) +DOB2C placed through the bit placed 50 ft above the casing shoe. The following procedures were used:

1) The sand was penetrated using 9-ppg mud until circulation was completely lost.

2) At this point the hole was drilled blind using sea water until all the sand was exposed.

3) Simultaneously, sea water was pumped into the annulus between the drillpipe and the open hole at 8 bbl/min to keep the top of the sand from kicking.

4) Once the sand was entirely exposed, the loss zone was sealed using sea water+DOB2C (1:2).

This case history describes the application of SW+DOB2C (1:2) to the fifth sand. Loss zones in the upper sands had already been sealed by a single application each.

When I came aboard the rig, the drilling engineer at the site had had a little bad luck. He had run an M+DOB and had plugged the drillpipe. Pulling the plugged drillpipe out of the kicking hole was bad enough. But when the DOB in the drillpipe was reached, it was blown all over the rig by a high wind. A light rain then covered all the rig surfaces with a rain-water DOB slick that was indescribably slippery. Needless to say, our reception by the drilling supervisor was less than cordial.

Even so, the first application of SW+DOB2C went like silk. A squeeze pressure of 1,250 psi was developed and held while the plug set. The loss zone was cured. This prompted the drilling supervisor to agree that SW+DOB2C had been effective and his cooperation was

69

100% after that, even though he still had some reservations in regard to drilling engineers.

A brief description of the application of 105 bbl of SW+DOB2C (1:2) to the fifth sand is given below:

Drilling proceeded from 7,546 to 7,644 feet. In this interval mud losses became complete and drilling was continued blind until some shale had been drilled. At this point, DOB2C was run with one variation from earlier jobs. As the DOB2C plug was being pumped down at 8 bbl/min, the annulus was kept full by pumping sea water into it at 14 bbl/min. The drillpipe rate was increased to 10 bbl/min (maximum rate for two Halliburton pumps) as the DOB2C reached the bit and the rams were closed. As soon as pressure showed on the annulus, the rates were adjusted to 4 bbl/min on the annulus and 8 bbl/min on the drill-pipe. A squeeze pressure of 1,250 psi developed, 1,150 held after pumping was stopped. Circulation had once again been restored, but it had been necessary to pump at a combined rate of 24 bbl/min, much higher than at any other time in our experience.

With the bit and collars still safely 50 ft above the casing shoe, SW+DOB2C was pumped 750 ft down the hole to plug loss zones in the sixth sand. The well was then drilled to total depth without further losses.

M+DOB2C Plugs are Permanent

Correctly formulated, M+DOB2C plugs develop from 500–1,150 psi of compressive strength at 180°F in 24 hours. They form permanent seals, so this property should be carefully considered before applying them to loss zones in productive formations.

Are Set M+DOB2C Plugs Hard Enough to Deviate Holes?

M+DOB2C plugs, as stated above, develop from 500–1,150 psi in 24 hours at 180°F. In my experience, this amount of strength has never been enough to deviate a hole. There have been reports of this occurring, however. There is nothing sacred about the cement-to-bentonite ratio in DOB2C. Lower the amount of cement in it if the formation taking mud is so soft that deviating the hole is likely.

Technique 5A—Mud + Diesel Oil-Attapulgite-Bentonite-Four Cement (M + DOAB4C)

Use M+DOAB4C where the water used in the mud to be used contains more than 10% salt. Also use it against water flows that contain more than 10% salt, particularly saturated brines containing magnesium, potassium, or calcium salts. The procedures for mixing and applying M+DOAB4C are the same as for M+DOB2C. Density and yield calculations for DOAB4C are given in Table 5–7.

TABLE 5–7   Density and Yield Calculations for DOAB4C

Volume of material, gal	Specific volume, gal/lb	Weight of material, lb	Material	Diesel-oil requirement, gal
4.15	0.0415	100	Attapulgite	
4.53	0.0453	100	Bentonite	53
14.36	0.0382	376	Cement	
		371	Diesel oil	
23.04 gal volume of solids		947-lb Weight of slurry		23.04
				76.04 gal volume of slurry

Slurry density, lb/gal, equals 12.45
Slurry yield, in cu ft/100-lb sack of attapulgite, equals 10.17
Bbl of slurry/bbl of diesel oil equals 1.44

Technique 6—Surface-mixed Soft Plugs

Use this technique against induced vertical fractures and to hold cements near the well bore where oil muds are used. Pal-Mix 100-R is a blend of synthetic polymers with auxiliary chemicals. This blend forms a time-delayed, self-complexed plug that is tough and insoluble when added to a suitable mix water. The plug is used as a temporary or permanent lost-circulation material. Also, it has application where water-base or oil-base muds are in use since it is surface mixed.

Pal-Mix 110-R can be mixed in fresh or sea water or in potassium or sodium chloride brines but not in calcium chloride brines. The plug can be weighted to 19.0 ppg with barite or iron carbonate. It is nontoxic, noncorrosive, and nonpulluting. A Pal-Mix 110-R plug can be reverted to its mix water at a predetermined time by incorporating a small amount of enzyme breaker.

Simplified safety-first mixing instructions for weighted Pal-Mix 100-R plugs are as follows:

1) Be sure the tanks are clean (for large plugs, a ribbon blender is very effective)
2) Use clean mix water or solution free of calcium ion
3) Raise pH to 10.0 with caustic soda—never over 12.0
4) To retard the plug, add Pal-Mix Xtender-B as needed for pump downtime

Hole depth, ft	Lb/bbl Xtender
4,000–9,000	3
9,000–11,000	4
11,000–13,000	5
13,000 and deeper	6

5) Add barite to the desired weight. Note: Water will not suspend barite satisfactorily without violent agitation. Do not attempt to mix the plug without adequate agitation.

6) Check and adjust the pH to 10 (9–11)

7) Check and make sure pumping crew and equipment are sitting on ready. This is very, very important.

8) Add 25–30 lb/bbl of Pal-Mix 110-R as fast as possible

9) Most important—as soon as the last bag of Pal-Mix 110-R is added to the plug, start pumping. Do not, *repeat,* do not shut down for anything. If a line breaks or other trouble develops, pump the plug on the ground. If this material sets up in your pipes or tanks, you will have trouble removing it.

10) Spot the plug into the loss zone and then shut down and wait on the plug for two hours.

Technique 7—Downhole-mixed Soft Plugs

Use this technique against induced fractures and to hold cement slurries at or near the well bore until they set.

The success of downhole-mixed soft plugs depends on having the right amount of the components meet and mix near the loss zone. Close attention should be paid to this. It is difficult to judge how much mud is going past the mixing sub when pumping into an annulus when it is not full. One can only be sure of the rate when the hole is full. When the hole is not full, mud should be pumped into the annulus early in the displacement of the plug in an attempt to fill the hole and thereby establish the optimum constant mud-flow rate at the mixing sub before the plug in the drillpipe leaves. Another complication is that the column of mud, diesel oil, and plug inside the drillpipe can be heavier than the mud in the annulus. It may fall and reach the mixing sub before all the mud required to put the diesel oil ahead at the mixing sub has been pumped.

The slurry density and yield calculations for diesel oil-bentonite (DOB) are given in Table 5–8.

TABLE 5–8   Slurry Density and Yield Calculations for Diesel Oil-Bentonite (DOB)

Volume of solids, gal	Specific volume, gal/lb	Weight of material, lb	Material	Diesel oil requirement, gal
4.53	0.0453	100	Bentonite	10.5
		73.5	Diesel Oil	
			(7 lb/gal)	4.53
		173.5		15.03
		weight of		volume of
		slurry, lb		slurry, gal

Slurry density, lb/gal, equals 11.54
Slurry yield, cu ft/100-lb sack of bentonite, equals 2.01
Bbl of slurry/bbl of diesel oil equals 1.43

*Soft plugs that are mixed at the surface have been differentiated from those mixed downhole because on many occasions Magcobar Form A Plug (surface mixed) has out-performed diesel oil-bentonite (downhole-mixed) even though diesel oil-bentonite correctly mixed will have better properties. It is difficult to mix two materials correctly in a hole that is losing circulation. Diesel oil-bentonite fails because, if it is too thick, it plugs the hole before reaching the loss zone and, if it is too thin, it will not plug the loss zone.

Technique 7—Diesel Oil-Bentonite (DOB) Bradenhead Squeeze [17, 18, 19]

Consider the following lost-circulation problem: 9⅝-in. casing had been set at 10,000 ft. One thousand feet of 8½-in. hole had been drilled below it when circulation was lost. A 10.0 ppg fresh-water mud was being used. Partial mud losses had occurred at 10,075 ft but had been sealed using bridging agents in mud (technique 2). When designing and applying an M + DOB squeeze:

1) Make sure all the lost-circulation zone is exposed. Run in to bottom to be sure there is no fill. If it is the first time the loss has been encountered, if possible drill without returns through the loss zone.

2) Locate the loss zone; determine its type and severity. (It is a severe induced vertical fracture at about 10,075 ft.)

3) Choose the right lost-circulation material and technique (DOB). Run pilot tests using the 10.0-ppg mud and 11.54-ppg DOB. From these choose a lead slurry (M+DOB (1:1.5)) and a final slurry (M+DOB (1:3)). See Fig. 5–13.

4) Choose an amount of DOB (20 bbl). It is assumed that the rig has a supply of bulk bentonite that can be delivered to the cementer's hopper.

5) Pull out of the hole. Put on a mixing sub consisting of 5 ft of appropriate-sized drillpipe orange-peeled at the lower end and a box

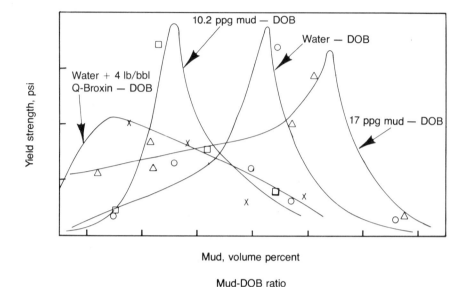

Fig. 5–13   Effect of mud-DOB ratio on final yield strength of mixture

end looking up and with 4 1-in. by 4-in. slots cut 1 ft above the end, as shown in Fig. 5–10. DOB can be placed through the bit if required, but because of the complications of the drill collars the danger of sticking the string is much greater.

6) Set the bottom of the mixing sub 50–150 ft above the loss zone (9,925 ft that, in this example, is up in the casing 75 ft). Install a 0–2,000-psi gauge on the annulus.

7) Set a maximum squeeze pressure (1,500 psi).

8) Place 20 bbl diesel oil in the cementer's tanks; pump 10 bbl diesel oil ahead. Somewhat lesser amounts can be used at shallower depths but not less than 5 bbl. Refill the tank with diesel oil.

9) Using bentonite from the bin and diesel oil across the hopper, hopper mix 27 bbl DOB into the drillpipe. Every bbl of diesel oil yields 1.43 bbl of 11.54-ppg DOB. The DOB could also be batch mixed if more convenient.

10) Pump 5 bbl diesel oil behind the DOB.

11) Displace the slurry down the drillpipe at 10 bbl/min with *airfree* mud. Slow the rate to 3 bbl/min when the diesel oil ahead reaches the mixing sub.

12) If there are no returns, simultaneously start pumping mud into the annulus at 2 bbl/min when the displacement of the DOB is started. Even if the hole fills and circulates (or if there are returns at the outset),

continue pumping into the annulus at 2 bbl/min. When the diesel oil ahead reaches the mixing sub, close the rams. This is to avoid pumping 10 bbl.of diesel oil up around the pipe. Diesel oil so placed would mix with the DOB instead of mud when the squeeze started, diluting rather than setting it.

13) Displace 15 bbl of slurry through the sub at this mixing rate. Lower the rate on the annulus to 1 bbl/min and increase the rate on the drillpipe to 3 bbl/min. This forms the final M+DOB2C (1:3) slurry. Pressure should build on the annulus at the end of step 12. Do not exceed 1,500 psi. By pumping at the slower rates, displace the plug 25 ft below the mixing sub.

14) Hold the squeeze pressure for 30 to 60 min. Open the BOPs and circulate and condition the mud to the desired properties and weight. M+DOB does not develop compressive strength. It may be so soft that it cannot be felt by the bit. Therefore, when drilling out drill rather than wash through all the plug. If the bit is run down through M+DOB, circulating the amount of M+DOB around the collars out may break down the loss zone again.

15) During the mixing, placement, and waiting periods, move the drillpipe occasionally to make sure it is free.

16) After conditioning the mud, pull out of the hole for a bit, drill out the plug, and then drill ahead. If no squeeze pressure develops, repeat the procedure using larger volumes or proceed to DOB2C (technique 5).

17) Check Fig. 5–11 for a pressure-chart summary of a squeeze.

Case History

An active lost-circulation zone was opened at 6,947 to 6,949 ft in a well in Western Canada. Seven-in. casing had been set at 6,603 ft. Sour (0.5 vol% H_2S) gas, from the interval 6,947 to 6,949 ft, pushed the mud from the hole, and in 30 minutes 3,000 psi pressure built up below the blowout preventers. Attempts to regain circulation and kill the well met with little success.

The well stood with drillpipe in the hole and 3,000 psi pressure on the preventers for a number of months until a workover rig could be moved in. When an attempt was made to break circulation, the drillpipe plugged. In trying to strip out of the hole, the drillpipe parted at 1,445 ft. It was decided that a successful fishing operation couldn't be carried out at 3,000 psi surface pressure. The next job was to establish circulation, to kill the well, to recover the fish and to run a packer and a production string of tubing. A diesel oil-bentonite (DOB) squeeze was selected to plug the loss zone.

The DOB squeeze was successfully applied to this very severe, active lost return zone as follows: The surface pressure was lowered from 3,000 psi to 800 psi by pumping water into the annulus. The well was then killed by pumping 10.2-ppg mud into the annulus behind the water. Just as the surface pressure reached zero psi, 20 bbl of DOB were pumped from the break in the drillpipe (at 2 bbl/min) and mixed with mud being pumped into the annulus (at 4 bbl/min). The 60 bbl of mud+DOB (2:1) formed was then pumped down the annulus between the fish and the casing so 6 bbl entered the loss zone and 54 bbl remained up around the fish. This plug restored circulation, whereupon the 10.2 lb/gal mud pumped behind the plug killed the well. The fish was then recovered, a production string run, and the well put onstream. Certainly this is a spectacular example of applying the right amount of the right material in the right place at the right rate.

The reason that M+DOB (2:1) was chosen over M+DOB2C is obvious. The object was to seal the loss zone and still be able to recover the fish without washing over. Since M+DOB develops high shear strength but does not set, its properties were superior to M+DOB2C, which also develops high shear strength but then sets. It is nice to have this positive situation where M+DOB clearly has the right properties. It is not very often that the more permanent M+DOB2C is not the first and best choice.

Given below is a refresher summary of mixing and placing DOB2C and DOB.

M+DOB2C and M+DOB (soft plugs) are materials that develop high shear strength rapidly when first mixed.* However, there is a difference between them; M+DOB remains plastic while M+DOB2C develops compressive strength much as cement does.

Example M+DOB2C Application

Problem: When complete circulation was lost, casing (9⅝-in.) had been set at 10,000 ft and 1,000 ft of 8¾-in. hole had been drilled using 10.0-ppg mud. Partial losses had occured earlier but were sealed using bridging agents in the mud.

Variables That Require Definition	Sample Situation
1. Determine type and severity of loss zone	1. Severe induced fracture
2. What is its location?	2. In shale within 300 ft of shoe
3. Choose lost-circulation material**	3. DOB2C
4. Method of placement	4. Bradenhead squeeze; diesel oil ahead and behind the DOB2C
5. Method of mixing	5. Batch mix in cementers tanks
6. Amount*** of 12.4-ppg DOB2C	6. 20 bbl

Variables That Require Definition	Sample Situation
7. Materials required	7. 14 bbl diesel oil (DO), 22 sacks bentonite; 44 sacks class-A cement
8. Set maximum annular squeeze pressure	8. 1,500 psi
9. Amount of DO ahead of the DOB2C	9. 10 bbl
10. Amount of DOB2C required	10. 20 bbl of 12.4 ppg
11. Amount of DO behind the DOB2C	11. 5 bbl

NOTE: If hole circulates during mixing, BOPs must be closed when DO ahead reaches bit or DO will come up around the DP.

12. Choose beginning total pump rate	12. 6 bbl/min
13. Choose mud to DOB2C ratio of lead (thin) M+DOB2C from the pilot tests run at the outset of the job	13. 1:1

NOTE: When DO reaches bit, close the BOPs and pump 3 bbl/min mud into both the DP and annulus

14. At 15 bbl DOB2C displaced, pressure reaches 1,300 psi	14. Change ratio to 1:2 (final slurry); lower total rate to 3 bbl/min— pressure falls to 1,000 psi
15. At 19 bbl, DOB2C displaced; pressure reaches 1,500 psi	15. Lower total rate to 1½ bbl/min; pressure falls to 1,300 psi (pump 1 bbl on DP; ½ bbl on annulus)
16. At 20 bbl DOB2C displaced; pressure reaches 1,500 psi	16. DOB2C completely displaced; hold pressure for 30 minutes; withdraw DP to safety; WOC 18 hours

*M+DOB and M+DOB2C are placed by bradenhead squeeze. DOB2C slurry is prepared in the cementer's tanks (or continuously hopper mixed) and then pumped down the drillpipe while mud from the rig tanks is pumped down the annulus. The two mix at the bit (or mixing sub), which should be placed just above the loss zone, and react to form a highly gelled mass that is then pumped down the open hole and into the loss zone.

**Briefly, M+DOB2C is used in preference to M+DOB against mud losses primarily to induced fractures and underground blowouts that are more severe. Other factors that may help with a choice between them are (1) M+DOB2C sets and require WOC time if its full value is to be realized; also it is more apt to stick the tools, (2) M+DOB develops most of its shear strength in an hour and, since it remains relatively soft, is less apt to stick the tools or cement off an access to the zone of interest.

***Amount of M+DOB2C depends on severity of the loss zone and hole size.

Technique 7A—Bengum

Halliburton's Bengum is a natural gum plus a preservative and complexing agent.[20] Bengum mix is 10 wt % Bengum No. 1 and 90% bentonite premixed together. Bengum slurry is prepared by adding 100 lb of Bengum-bentonite mix to 13–15 gal of diesel oil. Because of the organics it contains, it sets harder than DOB— particularly when mixed in saline waters and muds (Fig. 5–14). Its strength falls between that of DOB and DOB2C, but it is more nearly like DOB.

It should be used where more strength than that given by DOB is required and where saline mixing waters are significantly lowering the strength of DOB. For application, follow the instructions for DOB above. The recommended ratio of mud to Bengum varies from 4:1 to 1:1, according to the strength required. In areas where it is available, the use of Bengum should be considered.

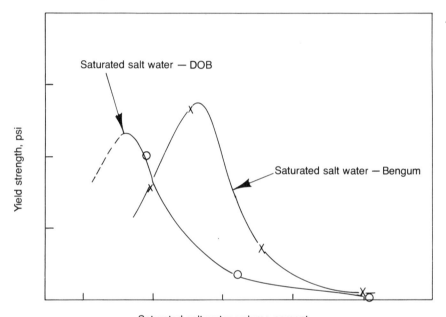

Saturated salt water, volume percent

Water phase to oil phase ratio

Fig. 5–14 **Effect of ratio of saturated salt water to DOB and Bengum on final yield strength of mixture**

Technique 7B—Polymer Plug

Dowell Polymer Plug is a 10:90 blend of polymer-bentonite slurried in diesel oil or other light oil. This blend of polymer and bentonite can be made up in bulk. Polymer Plug mixed with fresh or salt-water based drilling fluid results in the hydration of the polymer and bentonite. The putty-like mass formed as a result of hydration will give a nearly permanent plug in zones of loss.

Polymer Plug can be either continuously mixed with diesel oil or batch mixed. The density of the diesel-oil slurry can be varied from 8.3–

12.3 ppg. The recommended density is 10.5 ppg (300 lbs of blend per bbl of diesel oil). The yield is 1.3 bbl of Polymer Plug per bbl of diesel. Typical quantities per job of Dowell Polymer Plug would be 20–50 bbl with a 5–10 bbl spacer of diesel oil ahead and behind.

Polymer Plug should be applied as DOB is applied. It resembles Bengum in its strength development in that it develops greater strength than DOB particularly in saline waters and muds.

Technique 7C—Oil Mud-Water-Oleophilic Bentonite (OM + WOB)

M+DOB2C, M+DOAB4C, M+DOB, Bengum and Polymer Plug have little or no application where oil muds are in use because a water-base mud is an essential ingredient of these materials. However, there is a plug that is gelled by oil muds. Water-oleophilic bentonite (WOB) is such a plug. The composition and properties of various OM+WOB (1:1s) are shown in Table 5–9.

Mostly, WOB will be batch mixed. However, a dry blend of barite and oleophilic bentonite or oleophilic bentonite alone could be placed in a bin and hopper mixed into water containing the dispersant and the caustic if the need for large amounts of OB+WOB arose. WOB is placed in the same manner as DOB except that water (not diesel oil) is run ahead and behind it and it is mixed downhole by adding oil-base mud to it. WOB has no application where water-base muds are in use. I have never applied OM+WOB to a loss zone, so I can offer no first-hand experience.

On the average, OM+WOBs develop a maximum of 5–10 psi of shear strength. By comparison, M+DOB develops a maximum of 30–40 psi, and M+DOB2C develops a maximum of 45–60 psi. M+DOB2C then sets to develop compressive strengths of from 500–1,150 psi (see Figs. 5–6, 5–13, Table 5–9). Because of a possible strength deficiency, pilot testing OM+WOBs before a job is extremely important. If the oil mud in use was heavily weighted (16.0 to 18.0 ppg), then it could be possible that there would be no advantage to adding barite or other weighting material to the WOB in an effort to lower cost and increase shear strength.

Technique 7D—Hallibuton's Flo-Chek Process

Use this technique against severe complete losses to horizontal and vertical loss zones. The three-component system with cement-$CaCl_2$ has limited use against deeper, hotter induced vertical fractures unless it can be suitably retarded.

TABLE 5–9 The Composition and Properties of Oil Mud Plus Water Oleophilic Bentonite, OM+WOB (1:1s)

WOB Slurry Weight, lb/gal	11.3	11.0	10.1	12.4	11.6	11.0
Yield Strength for 50:50 Mix with Oil Mud, psi	1.7	8.4	1.6	1.3	2.3	7.0
WOB Slurry Volume, bbl slurry/bbl water	1.75	1.59	1.49	1.59	1.54	1.49
Mixing Water, bbl water/100 lb Oleophilic Bentonite	0.36	0.35	0.36	0.40	0.38	0.36
Oleophilic Bentonite (Geltone etc), lb/bbl water	274	284	280	248	261	275
Limestone, lb/bbl water	163	93	0	-	-	-
Barite, lb/bbl water	-	-	-	248	156	93
Q-Broxin, lb/bbl water	4.8	4.6	4.3	4.6	4.6	4.6
Caustic Soda, lb/bbl water	2.5	2.2	2.1	2.2	2.3	2.2

The Flo-Chek process can actually be three separate formulations:

1) Two-component system A—10% calcium chloride solution followed by Flo-Chek Chemical A or Injectrol A.

2) Three-component system—10% calcium chloride solution followed by Flo-Chek Chemical A or Injectrol A followed by a cement slurry + 2% calcium chloride (10% calcium chloride solution can be substituted for the cement).

3) Two-component system B—Flo-Chek Chemical A or Injectrol A followed by a cement slurry + 2% calcium chloride.

Flo-Chek Chemical A or Injectrol A are calcium ion-reactive liquids that form a highly gelled mass when contacted intimately with calcium ions. The source of the calcium ion can be (a) adding calcium chloride salt, (b) using a surface brine containing at least 6 weight % calcium chloride, or (c) from a brine that contains at least 6 wt % calcium in the formation to be treated.

Two-component system A forms a highly gelled mass that doesn't set and is similar to other downhole-mixed soft plugs. The three-component system forms a highly gelled mass on both the leading and the following edges of the calcium-reactive component, and the following cement then sets to make the seal permanent. As with other squeeze techniques, it is beneficial to hold any squeeze pressure that develops until the cement sets. Silica flour or 20–40-mesh sand and/or polypropylene fibers can be added to give bridging properties to the components before they are gelled.

Case History

I have had no first-hand experience with the Flo-Chek systems. Therefore, I can supply no case histories. However, Halliburton supplied the following:

Flo-Chek was applied to a 361-foot zone with complete lost circulation in a 12¼-in. hole while drilling at 15,280 ft.

Well Information:

Hole size:	12¼ in.
Drilling depth:	15,280 ft
Lost-circulation zone:	12,194–12,555 ft
Mud weight:	14.1 ppg
Drillpipe:	5", 19.50 lb

Job Procedure:

1. Ran radioactive tracer and temperature logs to determine zone
2. Pulled 12¼-in. bit to 10 ft above top of zone
3. Pumped 20 bbl fresh water to clean drillpipe and formation
4. Pumped 20 bbl 10% calcium chloride water
5. Pumped 5 bbl gelled fresh-water spacer
6. Pumped 50 55-gal drums Flo-Chek solution
7. Pumped 5 bbl gelled fresh-water spacer
8. Displaced with 14.1 ppg mud; rams closed
9. Pulled 500 ft drillpipe; circulate bottoms up
10. Circulate back through zone and drill ahead

The fresh-water spacer was gelled using 40 lb/bbl gel to minimize fingering through the heavy mud in the 12¼-in. hole.

Six additional jobs were run using the same procedure with the exception that the amounts of calcium chloride water and Flo-Chek were changed, depending on the number of feet taking fluid. Circulation was established on all jobs run and no zones took fluid later during drilling.

One job was run in an 8¾-in. hole where there had been a 7-ft fall of the bit. Attempts to regain circulation using cement were unsuccessful. Next, 3,000 gal of Flo-Chek followed by 300 sacks of class G cement containing 10 lb Okie #1 per sack were run. After waiting on cement and drilling out, the well was drilled to TD without any additional lost circulation.

The amount of material used on each job will vary due to fluid level and such. However, 100–200 gallons of Flo-Chek per foot of zone have been run, and on all jobs the calcium chloride water has been one-half the amount of Flo-Chek used. Positive surface squeeze pressures were obtained on all jobs except one by using the above procedures.

These case histories smack of success. Still, I have had as much— even greater—success running M+DOB2C, which is cheaper, more available, and no more complicated to mix and apply. Do not forget, however, that M+DOB2C has little or no application where oil muds are in use. All three Flo-Chek systems described above do have and should be considered strongly for this application. Again, two-component Flo-Chek system B (The calcium-reactive material followed by cement), according to Halliburton, has been successfully used to plug a lost-circulation zone by running it ahead of cement while cementing the casing. M+DOB2C cannot boast such an application. Therefore, Flo-Chek has a place in the drilling industry as a lost-circulation cure but should be used where the cheaper, more available, and comparably effective M+DOB2C has little or no application.

Technique 8—Specialized Agents (Water, Gelled Water, Gelled Oil-carrying Sand)

Use this technique against severe complete losses to induced vertical fractures and to losses to productive zones.

Water-carrying sand and gelled water-carrying sand were used to control a well kicking and losing sour gas. The situation at the well was so bizarre that it is best to start with the case history and then make a summary of who supplies the materials and how they are best mixed.

Case History

On December 3, 1975, with a 7-inch liner set at 3,193 m, a dolomite interval (3193–3283 m) in a well in Europe was tested and produced 50,000 cu m per hour of sour gas (19% H_2S, 19% CO_2). The zone, however, was not the final objective and, after careful consideration, a decision was made to drill by it without setting a second liner. Six-inch hole was drilled with 1.53 sp gr mud (pH–13.0) to 3,462 m where circulation was lost. The upper uncased sour-gas zone kicked. As the bubbles surfaced, all the mud was forced into the loss zone, leaving the hole full of sour gas. While a decision as to how to proceed was being made, the drillpipe parted at about 350 m.* Attempts were then made to kill the well with water and mud and to restore circulation with mud plus lost-circulation material to no avail. After the treatments, the well stood with 210–300 atm of sour-gas pressure on the pipe rams. A nearby creek was dammed up and water was pumped continuously while preparations were being made to sand-off the lost-circulation zone with 100 sacks of 10–20-mesh frac sand. Pumping the water had two desirable effects: (1) it reduced the surface pressure to 150 atm, and (2) protected the casing and drillpipe from the sour gas.

There was another complication: When the pipe rams were closed, they closed right under a tool joint; as the pressure built up, the drillpipe was pushed up through the rams, bending the kelly and drillpipe into grotesque S shapes. When the pressure was lowered, the drillpipe would go back into the hole. This sequence occurred eight times before the well was killed, the rams opened, and the damaged drillpipe and kelly replaced.

On December 16 the well was treated with 100 sacks of 10–20-mesh frac sand contained in 50 cu m of water. The mixture was displaced with 50 cu m of 1.45 sp gr drilling mud. The kill line was then opened and the well flowed dry sour gas after producing seven cu m of mud. The small volume of mud showed that the gas was now coming up through just the drillpipe and that the treatment had plugged the annulus between the drillpipe and casing above the active gas zone. Water was pumped into the well at a rate high enough to displace the gas into the loss zone and then pumped continuously at 1,000–1,500 liters/min.

At this point, the well was killed by pumping 1.80 sp gr mud; it could be kept dead by pumping 350 liters/min of drilling mud into the kill line. Opening the rams and replacing the damaged drillpipe and kelly under these circumstances was considered but decided against because, once opened, the rams might not have closed on the damaged drillpipe had the need arisen.

A decision was made to plug the loss zone using 15 to 20 pounds of 10–20-mesh frac sand per gallon of gelled water. This mixture was chosen over the sand-in-water mixture run earlier because the volume required (2 cu m compared to 50 cu m) was much less, thereby allowing it to be more nearly completely displaced with a full column of mud

---

*The mechanism involved here is stress corrosion cracking. Possibly it could have been prevented by placing the bit on the bottom of the hole and then slacking off weight equal to the weight of the collars. This would lower the stress on the drillpipe.

before possible sand-off. (If an early sand-off occured as in the other case, the drillpipe would be full of water.) Ten cu m of gelled water (pad) were prepared. To two cu m were added 50 sacks of 10–20-mesh frac sand. First, 4 cu m of pad were pumped; next, the 2 cu m of pad containing the sand; then, 2 cu m of pad and finally 30 cu m of 1.60 sp gr mud.* Near the end of the displacement the pressure rose from 0 to 120 atm; this pressure was held for two hours. The damaged drillpipe and kelly were replaced and the well was observed for two days. It was dead. Next, the drillpipe down to the collars was fished from the hole, and the open hole was secured with a bridge plug topped with cement just above the collars. The hole was then deviated and redrilled to its objective depth where a 5-inch liner was run and cemented. It was agreed that should the slightest complication arise, the well would be abandoned.

Before running the second sand treatment, the possibility of plugging the drillpipe and not the loss zone was raised, in which event it might not be possible to pump into the well without rupturing the casing. This risk was accepted. Once the fish was picked up by the overshot, the depth to which the drillpipe was open was determined by a wire line. It was found that all the sand was still in the drillpipe and none had entered the loss zone.

The gelled water to carry the sand was mixed on location. Halliburton supplied the gelled water and the frac sand for this job. Many companies supply these materials worldwide (Table 5–10).

Mixing

Gelled water, oil, and methanol-carrying sand can be mixed in two ways: batch mixed and using a frac truck.

Dowell uses a frac truck. The polymer is added to the water and the sand is added downstream of the pumps using a sand blender. The cross-linking agent and the breaker, if required, are added downstream of the sand.

B. J. Hughes Inc. has a slurry that is usually mixed with 15 lb of gravel per gallon of fluid carrier. A typical 10-bbl slurry will contain 250 gal of high-viscosity fluid and 3,800 lb of gravel, and it will weigh 13–14 ppg depending on the density of the fluid used.

Most jobs will be done by mixing 10-bbl batches of slurry. A mixing tank equipped with a screw is required. The base fluid and additives are

---

*The sp gr of the mud was raised to 1.60 (instead of the 1.45 used to displace the first job) to more nearly ensure the drillpipe would be killed after a sand-off.

TABLE 5-10 Gelling Agents for Water, Oil, and Methanol

Name of Supplier	Gelling Agent's Trade Name					
	For Water		For Oil		For Methanol	
	Gelling Agent	Breaker	Gelling Agent	Breaker	Gelling Agent	Breaker
B. J. Hughes, Inc.	Terre-Pack	Yes	Allo-Pack	Yes	Metho-Pak	Yes
Dowell	YF "G"	Yes	YF "GO"	J318	—	—
Halliburton	Hydropac	Yes	Slurry Pack	Yes	—	—
Petroleum Associates of Lafayette, Inc.	PAL-MIX 380A	Yes	PAL-MIX 240	Yes	—	—
Western	Westpack 1	Yes	Low Friction Frac	Yes	—	—
	Apollo Gel	Yes	Maxi-0-74	Yes	—	—

85

added to the tank with the screw turning. This gives a fluid with some viscosity. With the screw turning, the sand is added and the fluid complexed. Slurries with gravel concentrations as high as 20 ppg of fluid have been successfully mixed.

A skid-mounted centrifugal pump should be used to pump the slurry from the mixing tank to the triplex pumps. The centrifugal's suction should be kept as short as possible, less than 6 feet, and should be as large as possible, usually 4 inches.

The Terra-Pack, Terra-Pack II, Allo-Pack, and Metho-Pack fluids all show substantial friction-reducing properties; thus, friction pressure should present no problems. Each slurry can be pumped down the tubing at any desired rate (precautions should be taken to stay below fracturing pressure) until the slurry is within 2 bbl of the formation. The pumps should be slowed and the slurry squeezed into the formation at ½ bbl/min. The slow rate helps minimize the mixing of the formation sand with the pack gravel. Continue to pump the slurry until a sand-out occurs. Excess slurry is then circulated out of the tubing.

Technique 9—Drill Blind or with Aerated Mud and Set Pipe

Use this technique against very severe complete losses to caverns, large natural horizontal fractures, and long sections of honeycomb. In the case of very severe loss zones such as big caverns (with or without water movement) or long (500–1,000 ft) zones of honeycomb or fractures, drilling blind or with aerated mud through all the loss zone and then setting pipe is the only technique that can succeed. These methods are well understood by operations people.

There are some aids to drilling the aerated mud that are worth mentioning:

Jet Subs

Jet subs help support the mud column and release air in the upper hole. When placed in the drillstring, one is positioned just above the loss zone and the other 500–1,000 ft below the zone. They are sized so they will pass most of the air at 1,000 psi but only a small amount of the air-mud mixture. To establish circulation, air alone is pumped first to aerate the mud column above the loss zone. Then mud is gradually added to the air. This mixture stops part of the flow of air through the upper sub and activates the lower sub. Finally, as the amount of mud in the air-mud mixture is increased, air and mud come around the bit.

Concentric Drillpipe[21]

Here the amount of air required in a large hole can be cut down.

Macaroni String[22, 23]

A macaroni (1½-in.) string is run on the outside of the last casing string and opens into the casing 200–600 ft below the static mud level so circulation can be established with low-pressure air. A choke should be placed in the 1½-in. string and sized so air pressure equal to or greater than the weight of the mud column can be built up above the choke. This prevents slugs of air from entering the mud column.

Barite and Barite-in-Oil Plugs

Barite Plugs

Use barite plugs as an effective means of controlling active zones in wells while regaining circulation, searching for a transition zone, and tripping.

If an overpressured zone is encountered during drilling, the mud weight is built up and controls the kick. This is a straightforward, not overly dangerous procedure. However, many times after a kick has occurred, a situation arises where the well is kicking and losing circulation simultaneously or blowing out underground. It is extremely dangerous to carry out any operation with a well under these conditions.

Obviously, if a seal could be placed in the well bore between the active and lost-circulation zones, returns could be regained or casing run in relative safety. Barite plugs are an effective means of obtaining such a seal.

Composition and preparation. A barite plug is a slurry mixed using barite, a complex phosphate thinner, and water. It is mixed using cementing equipment, pumped in place through the drillpipe, and spotted in the bottom of the hole as near the active zone as possible. The bit—even a jet type—does not have to be removed.

The plug should be placed as soon as possible after opening an active zone and losing circulation.

Function. Barite plugs seal the well bore in four ways:

1) Due to their low viscosities and yield points, the barite can settle to form a solid plug in the hole.

2) Their high density increases the hydrostatic head on the active zone and helps hold it.

3) Due to their filter loss, they can dehydrate to form a solid plug of barite in the hole.

4) Their high filter loss also can cause the hole to slough and bridge itself. This could be accomplished by dehydration or settling of the barite plug.

Properties. Accordingly, the properties a barite plug should ideally have are high filter loss, high settling rate, and high density. The effects of phosphate thinners and pH on these properties are shown in Figs. 5–15, 16, and 17. The data show that sodium acid pyrophosphate (SAPP) concentration should be in the range of 0.2–0.7 lb/bbl for optimum barite settling. pH should be adjusted to 8–10 (about 0.25 lb/bbl of caustic soda). The data in Fig. 5–16 shows that adding SAPP lowers filter loss. This effect is believed to be due to increased barite settling. The volume of a 21-ppg barite plug for 100 bbl of settled plug is shown in Table 5–11. The slurry density and yield calculations for a 21-ppg barite plug are shown in Table 5–12.

TABLE 5–11   **Volume of 21-ppg Barite Plug for 100 bbl of Settled Barite Plug**

Slurry density, ppg	21.0	SAPP, lb	56
Slurry volume, bbl	152	Fresh water, bbl	80
Barite, sacks	1060	Caustic, est. lb	20

TABLE 5–12   **Slurry Density and Yield Calculations for a 21-ppg Barite Plug**

Volume of solids, gal	Specific volume, gal/lb	Amount of material, lb	Material	Water requirement, gal
2.84	0.0284	100	Barite	3.2
—	—	0.053	SAPP	
—	—	0.019	Caustic	
		26.66	Water	2.84
2.84		126.73		6.04
		Weight of slurry, lb		Volume of slurry, gal

Slurry density, lb/gal, equals 21.0
Slurry yield, cu ft/100-lb sack barite, equals 0.81

Barites vary throughout the industry. Difficulty in getting them to settle properly has been experienced. In most, if not all, cases precise adjustment of the pH has solved this problem. Pilot tests of forming a barite plug from the barite to be used should be run prior to opening potential active zones.

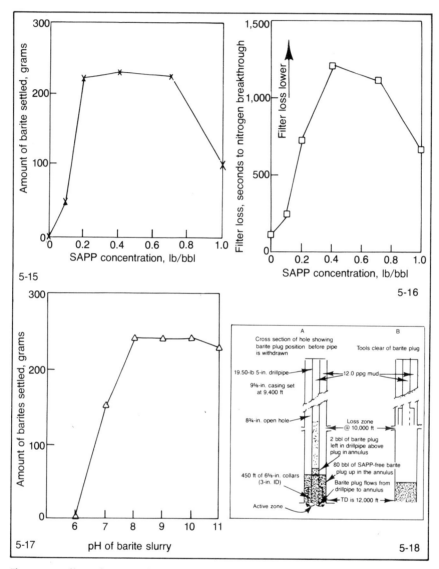

Fig. 5–15   Effect of SAPP on barite settled
Fig. 5–16   Effect of SAPP on filter loss of barite slurry
Fig. 5–17   Effect of pH on barite settled
Fig. 5–18   Placement technique

Barite plugs are best prepared in fresh water. Barite plugs, from which barite settles rapidly, have not been prepared using sea water. Accordingly, care should be taken to avoid the barite plug's being contaminated by saline formation waters or by any drilling mud during placement. Gas trickling through the plug is undesirable but not fatal. If there is an underground blowout of either gas, oil, or saline water, enough barite plug should be run to kill the active zone. Where long columns are run, SAPP should be added to the 450 ft in open hole and that which stays in the drillpipe. This limits the amount of unstable barite plug around the string and minimizes the danger of getting stuck. Where there is an active zone and circulation has been lost but no underground blowout is suspected, smaller plugs (usually 200–400 sacks of barite—enough to fill 200–450 ft of open hole and form at least 100 ft of settled barite plug therein) are often sufficient.

Case History

The example describes mixing and placing a barite plug large enough to kill the active zone. Consider the following hypothetical situation. An 8¾-in. hole was being drilled at 12,000 ft using 19.5-lb, 5-in. drillpipe and one foot of active zone was opened. The mud weight was increased from 11.0 to 12.0 ppg at this point, and circulation was lost to an induced vertical fracture at 10,000 ft.

Capacities:	bbl/ft
Collars	0.0087
Annulus between collars and hole	0.0317
Drillpipe	0.01776
Annulus between drillpipe and hole	0.0501
8¾-in. hole	0.0744

1) A slurry weight of 21 ppg is the correct choice for barite plugs. There is no use to complicate matters by using other weights.

2) It was decided that there was an underground blowout of gas and saline water to an induced vertical fracture at 10,000 ft. It was therefore necessary to kill the active zone with the barite plug. Enough should be run to reach the loss zone.

3) This would require enough SAPP-free barite plug to fill 1,550 ft of open hole (80 bbl is really 116 bbl, but 36 bbl will be in the drillpipe) and enough SAPP-treated plug to fill 450 ft of open hole (33.5 bbl + 36 bbl to fill the drillpipe). The SAPP-free barite plug should be mixed in clean, fresh water. The treated plug should be mixed in clean fresh water containing 0.7 lb SAPP/bbl with its pH adjusted to 9 with caustic soda (est. 0.25 lb/bbl).

4) Place the plug through the drillpipe as close to the active zone as possible.

5) Underdisplace the drillpipe so that the barite plug in the drill-pipe stands 2 bbl above the loss zone. To accomplish this, balance the columns as for cement plugs.

6) Pull 25 stands of drillpipe with the final position. This will put a 450-ft plug of SAPP-treated barite plug in the bottom of the hole and 1550 ft minus the displacement of the string of SAPP-free plug above it. Of course, as the drillstring is withdrawn, the SAPP-treated plug in the drillpipe will drain into the SAPP-treated plug in the bottom of the hole. It will also drain into the SAPP-free plug above it. This could cause barite to settle high in the hole but would not stick the drillpipe because the string stays above it.

7) Lighten the mud as much as feasible to restore circulation; circulate on top of the plug until the gas dissipates.

8) Go into the hole with the string with the pump off. If a firm plug is found at or below 11,900 ft, run casing.

The loss zone could be repaired using M+DOB2C, but it has already been demonstrated that the upper formations will not hold the weight required to control the active zone. Wash—do not circulate out—the barite plug to remove it. Attempting to circulate out 2,000 ft of 21.0-ppg barite plug will surely break down the loss zone again.

Barite-in-Oil Plugs

Use this technique where oil muds are in use against underground blowouts, where a well is simultaneously kicking and losing circulation, in searching for a transition zone, and for tripping. Barite-in-oil plugs can similarly be used with water-base muds.

The amount of barite-in-oil plug to run is 300 ft of settled plug in the open hole. Include a 10% excess to take care of hole enlargements if necessary. Enough volume of barite-in-oil plug should be run to hydrostatically kill the flow if the well is flowing downhole, as in an underground blowout.

Composition.   The mixture for each 100 bbl of settled barite from a 21.0-ppg barite-in-oil plug is shown in Table 5–13. Slurry density and yield calculations for it are shown in Table 5–14.

TABLE 5–13   Mixture for Each 100 bbl of Settled 21.0-ppg Barite-in-Oil Plug

Slurry volume, bbl	152
Barite, sacks	1060
Diesel oil, bbl	73.7
Oil-wetting dispersant 1, lb	300–450
Oil-wetting dispersant 2, lb	600

No. 1 dispersants are Magcobar's SE-11, Baroid's EZMul and Driltreat, Imco's Ken-thin, and Oil Base Inc.'s SA-27. No. 2 dispersants are Magcobar's Verthin and Milchem's Carbo-mul and Surf-Cote. These are effective, but it takes more of them to do the job.

TABLE 5–14 Slurry Density and Yield Calculations for a 21-ppg Barite-in-Oil Plug

Volume of solids, gal	Specific volume, gal/lb	Weight of material, lb	Material	Diesel oil requirement, gal
2.84	0.0284	100	Barite	2.92
		0.28	Dispersant	
—	—		Diesel oil	
		20.67		2.84
2.84		120.95		5.76
		Weight of slurry, lb		Volume of slurry, gal

Slurry Weight, lb/gal, equals 20.998
Slurry Yield, cu ft/100-lb sack barite, equals 0.77

Barite-in-oil plugs are mixed to weigh 21 ppg as are barite plugs in water with diesel oil substituted for the mixing water and oil-wetting dispersant substituted for the SAPP. They are placed in the same manner as barite plugs.

Case History

On March 4, 1974, while drilling a well in Canada at 10,711 ft using 8.5-ppg Invermul mud, circulation was lost and the well kicked. Circulation was reestablished using bridging agents-in-oil mud (technique 2); however, 1,800 bbl of mud were lost in the process. The mud weight was raised from 8.5 to 10.7 ppg. The increase in mud weight would appear to kill the active zone, but again it would kick. It was decided that casing should be run to control the kick for good, but it was felt that the well was kicking too much for casing to be run safely. A barite-in-oil plug was chosen to seal off the active zone prior to running casing.

On March 16, 24 bbl of winter diesel oil containing 2 lb/bbl of Baroid's EZMul were hopper mixed with 390 sacks of barite to form 50 bbl of barite-in-oil plug weighing 21.0 ppg. With the bit at 10,660 ft, the plug was pumped into the hole and was underdisplaced 6 bbl; 5 stands of drillpipe were pulled. (Barite settled from the surface samples, completely giving a solid plug ¾ of the original slurry in volume.) After two circulations above the plug, the well was completely dead.

The drillstring was started out of the hole preparatory to logging, but it stuck at about 5,400 ft with full circulation. The string had been in the hole for 14 days. Circulation was finally lost as the pipe was worked. The pipe was then backed off and the fish jarred loose and was recovered. The well remained completely dead during these operations.

After the fish was recovered from the hole, a conditioning trip was made prior to logging. With the bit at about 10,300 ft (above the top of Plug 1), the well was circulated. As bottoms came up, the well kicked, showing that after five days Plug 1 had broken down and the gas was bypassing it in some way. Plug 2 was then placed at 10,300 ft by operating personnel in the same way that Plug 1 had been mixed and placed. It consisted of 23 bbl of diesel oil containing about 2 lb/bbl of EZMul and 450 sacks of barite to give 54.4 bbl of 23.1-ppg slurry. This plug, as did Plug 1, shut off the gas. The 9⅝-in. casing was run 10,000 ft with full circulation and no gas; however, at 10,000 ft circulation was lost. Two joints of casing were washed into the hole to 10,080 ft without circulation. The casing was cemented at this depth. Just as mixing the cement was finished and displacement started, circulation reestablished and the annulus became active. The gas bubble was pumped out as the cement was displaced with full circulation; the annulus was dead at the end of the job. A cement bond log (CBL) showed good bonding with the top of the cement at about 7,200 ft—a 100% fill.

After drilling out, the shoe held 12.0-ppg mud equivalent and drilling proceeded using a 9.9-ppg Invermul mud.

CHAPTER 6
Special Situations and Lost-Circulation Problems

Controlling Water Flows

When drilling, encountering water flows from an active water zone to surface or from one zone to another in open hole or behind pipe is a common occurrence. Killing or controlling such water flows is, many times, a difficult and costly operation—if indeed they can be killed at all. It would be a safe to say many water flows go undetected. I have a deep-seated aversion to abandoning a well knowing that water (or any fluid for that matter) is flowing uncontrolled. Authorities in some countries demand that such flows be stopped. In West Germany, the Mining Authority has this responsibility.

Case History

During October, 1976, in West Europe while drilling a deviated hole at 4,678 m, a brine flow occurred and circulation was lost. Frac sand was applied to the loss zone, thought to be at bottom, and a sand-off was obtained. After the job, a temperature log showed there was no brine flowing from the bottom up the annulus to the weak (lost circulation) zones known to exist in the original hole at 2,620 m and 3,050 m. However, brine would flow from the well to the surface in large amounts (2,400 m^3). At first it was thought that, where the flow first occurred, it was from the second hole and the flow charged the upper weak zone in its two days of flow before the bottom was sanded off, so they could produce 2,400 m^3 of brine to surface. There is a possibility that there never was a brine flow or a loss zone in the second well. Rather, brine pressure built up in the first hole. When the mud weight in the second hole was raised to 2.24 s.g., the hole broke down at 3,050 m and the fracture extended into the first hole. Brine then flowed from the first hole to the second, causing another loss zone at 2,620 m and parting the drillpipe at 4,080 m, 1,265 m, 1,121 m and possibly the 13⅜-in. casing at 1,300 m.

In attempts to shut off the brine flow, various applications of frac sand, Pozmix 140 (pozzolan-lime cement), and Magne-Set (magnesia) cement were made without results. On November 6, it was decided to treat the well using diesel oil-attapulgite-bentonite-four cement

(DOAB4C), a brine and brine-mud reactive, in an attempt to kill the brine flow at surface.

At this point, a string of 13⅜-in. casing had been set at 2,539 m and cemented to a height of 893 m; 12¼-in. hole had then been drilled to 4,678 m in the deviated hole. The drillstring was in the hole with the bit at 4,619 m. The drillpipe was parted at 1,121 m and 1,265 m, and possibly there was a break in the casing at 1,300 m. There were also loss zones at 2,620 m and 3,050 m, both charged with brine from Well 1 and the latter containing gas.

At a meeting with the partners on November 6, it was decided to apply DOAB4C down the annulus from the break at 1,121 m in an effort to plug the possible casing leak at 1,300 meters and the annulus below it so that the drillpipe string could be repaired and access again established to lower troublesome zones through it. Accordingly, on November 7, 75 m³ of 2.24 s.g. mud were circulated at 500 m/min into the well down the drillpipe (casing 60, dp 100 bar). Both the casing and drillpipe held 100 bar when pumping was stopped. Another test was made with 3 m³ of mud at 500 1/min; casing 120, drillpipe 140 bar. Both held 100 bar. Next, 3 m³ of diesel oil, 10 m³ of DOAB4C (1.46 s.g.)*, 1.5 m³ diesel oil, and 22.5 m³ mud (2.24 s.g.) were pumped down the drillpipe, out of the break at 1,121 m, then down the annulus and possibly into the open formation through a break at 1,300 m. Squeeze pressure began at about 150 bar and rose to 280 bar as the last 10.5 m³ of displacement mud was pumped. By this application of DOAB4C, the annulus, drillpipe, and break in the casing at 1300 m were definitely plugged. With the well now dead, the breaks in the drillpipe were repaired and the drillpipe was washed free of obstructions with a Dynadrill on coiled tubing to 4,000 m.

Materials and Methods for Killing Water Flows

The following procedure should be followed:

1) Run a temperature survey to determine if brine (or fresher water) is flowing.

2) If there is flow, perforate the pipe in the appropriate place.

3) Establish an injection rate with mud.

4) Run a second temperature survey to determine where the flow is entering the upper formations.

5) If the flowing water is a brine, apply DOAB4C; if it is relatively fresh, apply DOB2C. Each of these must be applied at a rate that is twice

---

*Contained 5 t class g, 1.75 t bentonite, 1.75 t swdc (attapulgite) and 7,000 1 diesel oil.

as fast as the estimated rate of the flow until a squeeze pressure develops. If the flow is so fast that a 1:2 water to DOAB4C ratio cannot be obtained, attempt to slow it down by running a SAPP-free barite plug ahead. Clear the perforations and repeat the job if no squeeze pressure develops.

6) Run a third temperature log to find the top of the brine + DOAB4C (1:2) plug.

Method Mechanisms

By applying DOAB4C or DOB2C at the right rate, one can change a flowing brine or water into a highly gelled cement that impedes and then stops the flow. It then sets to make the seal permanent. These materials, as evidenced by the example, have been very effective in stopping water flows. For these plugs to be effective, though, a ratio of brine or water to DOAB4C or DOB2C of 1:2 must be obtained.

If the brine that was flowing happened to contain 6–10 wt % of calcium chloride, then the two-component Flo-Chek system B (Flo-Chek Chemical A or Injectrol A followed by cement) would be a good alternative choice, particularly if these materials could be delivered at higher rates.

Control of Water Flows during Cementing– A Case History

In a well drilling offshore North Africa 20-in. casing had been set at 813 ft. A 17½-in. hole was being drilled at 1,529 ft when a 256-bbl/hr water flow was encountered. Drilling 17½-in. hole proceeded to TD at 3,030 ft, allowing the annulus to flow and using sea water down the drillpipe for the drilling mud. The 13⅜-in. casing was run with a DV-tool at 1,529 ft and cemented in two stages.

The first stage consisted of 1,098 sacks of class G cement mixed in saturated salt water at 16.3 ppg. The cement column reached the active salt-water flow, which was 150 bbl/hr after the 13⅜-in. casing had been run. The DV tool was opened and the first-stage cement allowed to set as the annulus flowed.

The second stage was cemented with 700 sacks of class G cement plus 2% calcium chloride mixed in sea water at 15.8 ppg. This was followed in intimate contact with 10 bbl of diesel oil and 200 sacks of cement plus 25% brine gel and 25% bentonite mixed in diesel oil to weigh 12.4 ppg. Five bbl of diesel oil were run behind. This application reduced the water from 150 bbl/hr to 4.5 bbl/hr, whereupon 200 sacks of class G cement were bullheaded down the 20-in. by 17½-in. annulus to complete the seal.

Curing Mud Losses to Productive Zones
The Best Permeability is Always Sealed First

Whatever lost-circulation material is applied and whether it makes a temporary or permanent seal, it always enters and plugs the most permeable sections of the productive zone first. Accordingly, there is a desperate need in the drilling industry for a lost-circulation material and technique that is effective against mud losses to productive zones but, once the drilling and completion operations are over, leaves the productive zones undamaged.

Let's review the nine lost circulation techniques in terms of what permanent damage they may do to a productive zone. It takes only a cursory look to conclude that techniques 2–7 and particularly 3A through 7 do complete and permanent damage to productive zones. Only technique 1 (pull up and wait), technique 8 (gelled water or gelled oil carrying sand or sized crushed limestone) or technique 9 (drill blind or with aerated mud and set pipe) have any potential for being nondamaging to productive zones.

Temporary Plugging Agents

Technique 8, though still specifically untried as a nondamaging temporary plugging agent for productive zones, deserves consideration. Recall that all the gelled water and gelled oil systems can be treated with breakers to make them temporary. Also, they can carry sand or crushed limestone that could sand-off in the loss zone, propping it open and leaving a seal that mud-carrying bridging agent would not enter but that formation fluids would readily flow from. Sized limestone could be removed by acid, possibly restoring the best permeability in the productive zone to its original state. Definitely, programs to develop materials and techniques for curing mud losses to producitve zones should be given high priority.

Lost Circulation during Cementing

In my experience, lost circulation during cementing has not been a very serious problem. Yet it is highly desirable to have a complete cement sheath around the casing that is well bonded to both the pipe and the formation. This is often difficult, if not impossible, to do where there is no circulation prior to cementing or circulation is lost during cementing. Sections of hole are often drilled blind using sea or other water and the casing is only partially cemented, leaving the casing exposed to corrosive waters that literally dissolve it.

Prevent or Cure Lost Circulation before Cementing

Prevent it! Easier said than done? Not always. Establishing a stabilized circulation rate and then adhering to it whatever the operation in the hole will go a long way in preventing lost circulation. Given a stabilized hole and one is about to run casing, how should one proceed? Simply run the casing, circulate prior to cementing, mix, and displace the cement at the stabilized rate. This prevents pressure surges that will break down exposed weak formations and also prevents stirring up trouble in dirty, out-of-gauge, unstable holes.

Cure it! Locate the loss zone, define it in terms of type and severity, then match the lost circulation material and technique functionally to the type and severity and apply it in the right amount at the right rate in the right place. Choose from techniques 1 through 9.

The Nasty Loss Recurs during Cementing

Bridging agents can be added to the cement slurry itself when cementing holes that have had a prior history of lost circulation as an added means of prevention. Treat the cement slurry with 5 lb gilsonite/94-lb sack of cement or 6¼ lb of Kolite (ground coal). Ground black walnut hulls, peach pits, or olive pits can be substituted. Use a blend of 3 coarse, 2 medium, and 1 fine. Amounts larger than these may bridge at the collars or plug the float equipment. These amounts of granular agents seem to outperform small amounts of fine cellophane flake.

Lightening the cement slurry is a step in the right direction. However, heavier slurries and slurries lightened using hollow spheres, because of their high content of relatively coarse solids, have more self-sealing action than slurries lightened using bentonite, attapulgite, and silicates and water. For example, densified class G cement (16.5 ppg) has shown self-sealing properties when run to cement liners in deep, hot holes. Slurries lightened by hollow spheres, while limited to a depth of 6,000 ft, would exhibit similar properties. A DV tool could be run just above the potential loss zone.

But how should one proceed if circulation is lost while running casing, even though casing is being run correctly? Do not attempt to seal the loss by applying techniques 2 through 8 prior to cementing. Add bridging agents to and lighten or densify the cement slurry for a one-pass run at the loss zone. Also, there is evidence that the 2-component Flo-Chek slurry B can be effective. Run a fresh-water flush, then the Flo-Chek chemical A or Injectrol A solution, then more fresh-water flush, and finally cement slurry-2% calcium chloride and retarder as required. Here, all the calcium ion active material enters the loss zone where summarily it is contacted by the cement slurry. A highly gelled mass forms that seals the loss zone and restores circulation of the cement slurry up the annulus. No complication should arise in the annulus now since all the calcium ion reactive material is safely sealed in the loss zone. If there are two successive loss zones, run two Flo-Chek plugs ahead (if you're brave enough).

Well Losing Circulation and Kicking Sour Gas

There have been two instances in my career where I was confronted with a well that was losing circulation and kicking sour gas. One gas contained 0.5 vol % H_2S; the other 19.0 vol %. The dry sour gas pressure on the BOPs of the first well was 3,000 psi; on the second, it was 300 bar, which doesn't sound very high until you multiply it by 15. In the first well, the active and loss zone was a 2-ft natural fracture; in the other well, open hole had been drilled below an active zone and then circulation had been lost.

The approved procedure when circulation is lost is to pull the string off bottom immediately to prevent it from sticking. Actually, not doing this could be grounds for dismissal. This procedure is fine when the well does not fill with dry, sour gas. If it does and the bit is off bottom with the full weight of the collars on the upper section of drillpipe, the drillpipe may break due to stress corrosion cracking and the fish will stick on the bottom.

Stay On Bottom—Slack Off

When this situation arises, the bit should immediately be placed on bottom and at least the weight of the collars slacked off. This takes stress off the upper sections of drillpipe and lessens the danger of drillpipe failure due to stress-corrosion cracking. In both wells, the pipe parted at about 1,500 ft.

Pump Water—Any Water

The next precaution is to pump any available water as soon as possible. If water can be pumped at a sufficient rate, it serves two useful purposes: (a) it displaces all the H_2S-bearing gas into the loss zone and thus protects the drill string from it, and (b) it lowers the pressure on the BOPs by a significant and friendly amount. In the first well, the surface pressure was lowered from 3,000 to 800 psi. That's water pressure.

Now Cure the Loss

Once on a location, I was asked to go start a motor. As I approached it, I saw a sign with the word SEX in big red letters. After that was the phrase, "Now that I've got your attention, please check the oil, water, and fuel before starting this motor."

Now we have access to the loss zone instead of having the drillpipe parted and a fish stuck in the hole. Can you stand it once more? *Locate the loss zone, define it in terms of type and severity, match the material and technique functionally to its type and severity, and then apply them.*

Drill the Highest Mountain

Severe lost returns usually develop in holes drilled from mountain sites in the upper parts of the hole. The locations are often remote, inaccessible, and difficult and expensive to prepare. One advantage though—it is not often that the driller can locate the loss zone by looking from the rig floor down the mountain and observing where the mud is flowing from it.

It may be just coincidence, but oftentimes the access road traverses a valley before it starts up the mountain. A well drilled directionally from the valley floor might prevent the problem with lost returns.

Impossible-to-Plug Loss Zones

Make no mistake, there are some loss zones that are impossible to plug. A Carlsbad cavern, for instance, would be best drilled blind and then pipe set (technique 9).

In the Mideast to improve rig performance, a drilling game was initiated. All rigs were placed in direct competition and awards were given to the rig that drilled the fastest—not necessarily the cheapest and the best. Nonetheless, the game did sort out the best rig—the crew that would first plan a sound, detailed drilling program and, working together, would carry it out to the letter having anticipated problems and delays. For example, blame for the lack or delay of necessary services and supplies was not put on the service companies but was kept squarely on the rig's shoulders. But the clincher was that this rig was drilling in loss zones that had been impossible to plug for 30 years.

How does one approach an impossible-to-plug loss zone? In anticipation of this case, 4,000 96-lb sacks of B2C blend were mixed onshore. Of these, 2,000 sacks were placed in the rig's cement bins and 2,000 were kept alongside on the supply boat. In one of the rig's mud tanks, 450 bbl of 10¢/gal diesel oil were placed.

Once the 13⅜-in. casing had been set, the practice in the area was to drill the 12¼-in. hole the fastest possible way using sea water.

100

When circulation was lost, the loss zone would flow foul water that was deflected into the sea while sea water down the drillpipe was used for drilling. The 9⅝-in. casing was then run and cemented without circulation.

The best rig was about to start this sequence when it decided to attempt to prevent lost circulation by drilling with good mud at a controlled rate and really locate the impossible-to-plug loss zone. A mud with ideal flow properties and weighing 78 lb/cu ft (enough to give a 50-psi overbalance on the foul water-loss zone) was chosen. It was agreed that the crew would drill at a controlled rate with the mud, the properties of which would be meticulously maintained. The best rig never missed a trick and drilled past all the impossible-to-plug loss zones without losing even one barrel of mud. Then the 9⅝-in. casing was run and cemented to surface still without any mud losses.

The next assignment was impossible-to-plug loss zones in 3000 ft of 17½-in. hole. Unlike the first well, this well encountered successively very severe complete-loss zones. The procedure to plug them was first to drill 500 ft of hole blind using sea water. Next, DOB2C was sprayed using mixing sub A (see Fig. 5–11) into the sea water in the open hole converting it to M (sea water) + DOB2C (1:X). After this operation with the bit raised to a point just above the plug, a bradenhead squeeze of DOB2C down the drillpipe and sea water down the annulus was applied until 50–100 psi showed on the annulus. Of course the SW+DOB2C (1:2) was then allowed to set for 18 hours, whereupon the set SW+DOB2C plug was drilled out and the next 500 ft of hole were similarly drilled and treated. Using these materials and techniques, the well was drilled to casing depth. It was not easy, but at TD there was complete circulation before casing was run. Astoundingly, not a single pound of bridging agents was added to the mud; as a matter of fact, none was ever on location. By applying SW+DOB2C with this added dimension, these impossible-to-plug loss zones were holding clean mud.

Locate the loss zone, define it in terms of type and severity, then apply the right amount of the functionally right material at the right rate in the right place and even these impossible-to-plug loss zones could be and were plugged.

Any Barite Plug with Any Mud

Even though it may have been mentioned before in the section on barite plugs, it is worthwhile to highlight that any barite plug can be used with any mud. There appears to be no valid reason why barite plugs cannot be used where oil muds are in use or why barite-in-oil

101

plugs cannot be used where water-base muds are in use. The effectiveness of barite plugs is lowered if they are contaminated by drilling mud or formation brines or if gas is flowing through them. If a barite-in-oil plug rather than a barite plug were run where water-base mud was in use, the barite-in-oil plug would be more difficult to contaminate with drilling mud and formation brines. Also, up to saturation, flowing gas would be dissolved. On the face of these considerations, barite-in-oil plugs may well outperform barite plugs where water-base muds are in use.

The Added Dimensions of Lost-Circulation Control

The lost-circulation materials and techniques described in this book have more than one dimension. Below, the added dimensions of the right amount of the right material at the right rate in the right place are discussed, having chosen M+DOB2C as the right material.

The right amount. The right amount of M+DOB2C would give the sought-for squeeze pressure just as the M+DOB2C (1:2) plug, run from up in the casing, is displaced 25 ft below the mixing sub or the bit. The amount is chosen on the severity of the loss zone, experience, and luck, with too little preferable to too much. The right amount has at least three dimensions.

The right material. The right material is M+DOB2C (1:X). The mud can be any water-base mud—a dimension indeed. This is why the pilot tests with the mud in active use at the rig are so important. These tests should sort out two more dimensions; the ratio of mud to DOB2C for the lead slurry (1:1) and for the final slurry (1:2). Earlier, the ratio of 1 100-lb sack of bentonite to 2 94-lb sacks of cement was chosen on the basis of field performance. The standard DOB2C slurry weighs 12.4 ppg, but it could have many more dimensions. In summary, there are three dimensions of an M+DOB2C that must be defined: a) DOB2C is standard, b) the amount of mud for the lead slurry, and c) the amount of mud for the shoe slurry.

The right rate. The right total rate for 5-in. drillpipe in 8¾-in. and larger holes has been chosen at 8 bbl/min on the average. This is cut in half twice as pressure builds to get all the right amount of DOB2C away before the sought-for squeeze pressure is reached. Also, there are the rates of mud down the annulus and the drillpipe for the lead slurry and the final slurry. It is accurate to conclude that there are at least six rate dimensions required for a perfect job.

The right place. Here perhaps there is only one dimension proximate enough to the loss zone (preferably from up in the casing shoe) so the lead slurry can seek and plug the loss zone. But there is another dimension if the loss zone cannot be reached from the shoe and one must venture out into the open hole.

Whether the lost-circulation material and technique be M+DOB2C mixed and placed by bradenhead squeeze or any of the other techniques presented, for them to perform up to their full potential one must consider all their dimensions in the choice of the material and the method in which it is applied.

Prevent Lost Circulation during Leak-off Tests

A new procedure for leak-off tests in oil muds has been developed. Oil-base spacer suitably weighted (Baroid's EZ-Spot, for example) is spotted around the shoe. It stays in place, and its HTHP filter loss is 15 to 30 times more than that of an oil mud in good condition. This amount of filter loss appears to be enough for conventional leak-off.

Once a production string of casing has been set, the common practice is to first test the casing, then drill out the shoe, and finally drill about 30 ft of new hole. At this point, the integrity of the shoe is tested by running a leak-off test. The test should be up to leak-off pressure or the sought-for pressure, whichever is reached first. Fracturing pressure should not be exceeded.

Many times the shoe is broken down and a fracture is created. With water-base mud in use, the fracture has a finite chance to cure itself. But when oil-base mud is in use (and since fractures in oil mud are not self-repairing), added care needs to be exercised so the formations just below the shoe are not fractured.

Leak-off is easy to get and see where water-base muds are in use. But with oil muds in good condition, leak-off does not occur; the formation fractures before leak-off. To overcome this, water-base mud or diesel oil have been spotted across the shoe so there is a fluid that has enough filter loss there to leak off. This procedure is not the best because water-base mud contaminates the oil mud while diesel oil, being lighter, is apt to migrate from the shoe with predictable results.

APPENDIX A

API Specifications of Bridging Materials for Regaining Circulation

Equipment

10.1 The following equipment is used in testing bridging materials used for regaining circulation (see Fig. 10.1 and 10.2):

a. One set of ¼ in. (6.4 mm) thick by 1⅞ in. (47.5 mm) diameter stainless steel disks. These disks have square-edged slots 1⅜ in. (35 mm) in length and widths of 0.04 (1.0), 0.08 (2.0), 0.12 (3.0), 0.16 (4.0), and 0.20 (5.0) in. (mm).

b. One sleeve 2⅞ in. (73 mm) in diameter, 2¼ in. (57 mm) high with perforated base plate containing approximately thirty-two ¼ in. (6.4 mm) holes.

c. About 95 brass or stainless steel marbles ⁹⁄₁₆ in. (14.3 mm) in diameter (enough to just fill bed volume).

d. Approximately 1200 grams of brass-clad or stainless-steel BB shot [0.173 in. (4.39 mm) diameter] and a 10-mesh stainless-steel screen 2⅞ in. (73 mm) in diameter.

10.2 Additional equipment used in testing bridging materials is:

a. Source of pressure regulated nitrogen.

b. One graduated 3500-cm³ plastic container with inlet and outlet suitable to accommodate the sudden discharge of mud from the cell.

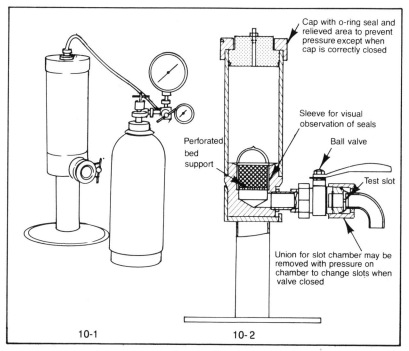

Fig. 10–1   Bridging material test equipment
Fig. 10–2   Bridging material test cell, 1,000 psi (70.3 kgf/cm²) working pressure

Procedure

10.3 Prepare a base mud consisting of 5 to 8 percent by weight Wyoming-type bentonite which has been aged a minimum of 72 hours and which has been adjusted to have an apparent viscosity of 25 centipoises ±2 centipoises after stirring 10 minutes on a multi-mixer.

10.4 To 3500 cm³ (10 laboratory bbl) of the base mud, add a weighed amount of the material to be tested. The additive concentration is expressed in lb per bbl.

Static Slot Test

10.5 Select a disk, preferably having a small slot, and place it in the valve outlet half-union with the perforated plate and sleeve used to support BB or marble beds removed from the cell. Open the cylinder bleed valve to the atmosphere and place the graduated container under the outlet.

10.6 Pour the mud containing the material to be tested into the cell with cell outlet valve open. Record the volume of mud which flows out. Screw the cap on the cell.

10.7 The free piston may be placed on the mud in the cell, if desired. Start the timer and apply pressure at a rate of 2 psi per second (0.14 kgf per cm² per second), until a pressure of 100 psi (7.03 kgf per cm²) is reached. Record the volume of mud discharged. The minimum pressure at which a seal occurs may or may not be observed: if observed, it should be recorded.

10.8 Increase pressure at a rate of 10 psi per second (0.7 kgf per cm² per second) to 1000 psi (70.3 kgf per cm²), or until the seal fails and the cylinder empties. Record the volume through or the maximum pressure obtained. If a seal is obtained, maintain the pressure for 10 minutes and record the final volume.

10.9 Repeat the test with increasing sizes of slots until no permanent seal is achieved at 1000 psi (70.3 kgf per cm²).

Dynamic Slot Test

10.10 Prepare base mud as described in Par. 10.4 and apparatus as outlined in Par. 10.5.

10.11 With the outlet valve closed, pour the test mud into the cell. The free piston may be placed on top of the mud. Close the cap and set the gas regulator to deliver at the test pressure, 100 psi (7.0 kgf per cm²). Open the cell outlet valve and start the timer. Record the volume of mud which flows through the slot and the time required to seal. Pressure can then be increased to 1000 psi (70.3 kgf per cm²), at the rate of 10 psi per second (0.7 kgf per cm² per second) and maintained for 10 minutes as in Par. 10.8

10.12 Repeat the test with increasing sizes of slots until no permanent seal is achieved.

Static Marble Bed Test

10.13 Prepare the marble bed by pouring the ⁹/₁₆-in. (14.3 mm) marbles into the sleeve so as to form a bed 2¼ in. (57 mm) thick above the perforated plate (just to the top of the container). Place the full-bore ring in the slot groove.

10.14 With the cell outlet valve open and a graduated container under the outlet, pour the test mud into the cell, and record the volume through the bed under the hydrostatic head.

10.15 Place the free piston on top of the mud and the cap on the cell. Close the cylinder bleed valve and start the timer. Apply pressure and record results as in Par. 10.7 and 10.8.

10.16 On completion of the test, release the pressure. Remove the marble bed and examine the appearance of the seal and the depth of penetration of the sealing material.

Dynamic Marble Bed Test

10.17 Prepare the marble bed as in Par. 10.13.

10.18 With the cell outlet valve closed, pour untreated base mud into the cell to fill the void spaces under and within the marble bed until the top of the untreated mud is level with the top of the sleeve.

10.19 Carefully pour the test mud into the cell so as not to disturb the mud in the bed. The free piston may be placed on top of the mud. Close the cell and apply pressure with the gas regulator adjusted to 100 psi (7.0 kgf per cm^2). Open the cell outlet valve and start the timer. Record the volume of mud which flows through the bed and the time to obtain a seal.

10.20 Continue the test as in Par. 10.8. After 10 minutes at 1000 psi (70.3 kgf per cm^2) or after failure, inspect the bed as in Par. 10.16.

Static BB Bed Test

10.21 Prepare the BB shot bed by placing the 10-mesh stainless-steel screen on the perforated plate and pouring the brass-clad or stainless-steel BB shot into the sleeve so as to form a bed 2¼ in. (57 mm) thick above the screen (just to the top of sleeve). The thickness of the shot bed can be varied from a minimum of 1 in. (25 mm) to 2¼ in. (57 mm). If less than 2¼ in. (57 mm) record the thickness. Place the full-bore ring in the slot groove. With the cell outlet valve open and the graduated container under the outlet, pour the test mud into the cell.

10.22 Proceed with the test according to Par. 10.14, 10.15 and 10.16.

Dynamic BB Bed Test

10.23 Prepare the shot bed as in Par. 10.21.

10.24 With the cell outlet valve closed, pour untreated base mud into the cell to fill the void spaces under and within the shot bed until the top of the untreated mud is level with the top of the sleeve.

10.25 Proceed with the test according to Par. 10.19 and 10.20.

APPENDIX B

Environmental Impact of Lost-Circulation Materials

For a book on lost circulation in drilling to be complete, not only must prevention and cure be part of it but also the effects of the materials and techniques on the environment and their effectiveness where both water-base and oil-base muds are in use. Their effectiveness where both water base and oil muds are in use is covered in detail in the text.

All of the lost circulation materials described in this book have been in active use by the drilling industry for years. They have either been classified as nondamaging or special treatments have been devised to render them nondamaging before they are disposed of on the land or in the seas and streams. Even though the rules vary widely worldwide, the drilling industry has made every reasonable effort to follow them and thus protect the environment to the fullest possible degree.

The hazard to the environment from lost-circulation materials is diminished even more because they are always applied downhole to a thief zone. By far, most of the loss agents and the vehicles that carry them are lost into the thief zone and never see the ecology again.

In the text of this book, a question in regard to the effect of loss agents containing diesel oil is raised. The reason is that while diesel oil is not really poisonous, even in minute amounts, it has a very objectionable taste and odor. Therefore, loss agents containing it should not be applied to formations bearing potable waters except in cases of extreme emergency, such as stopping an uncontrolled flow that would deplete the aquifer. Happily, water sands occur at rather shallow depths and losses to them are easily cured by agents free of diesel oil.

It is correct to conclude that, with the few precautions related above, the lost-circulation materials described in this book are not and will not be harmful to the environment or ecology.

REFERENCES

[1]Howard, G. C., and P. P. Scott, Jr., "An Analysis and the Control of Lost Circulation," Trans. AIME, 1951, p. 171.

[2]Glenn, E. E., Jr., and R. Jenkins, "Lost Circulation—A New Fibrous Material for its Correction," *Petroleum Engineer*, October 1951.

[3]Wilson, W. H., "Sawdust and Rice Hulls as Supplements to Leather Floc in Preventing Lost Returns," unpublished report, Mobil Research and Development Corp., Dallas, May 1955.

[4]Wilson, W. H., "Lost Returns Additives—Evaluation Tests," unpublished report, Mobil Research and Development Corp., Dallas, December 1955.

[5]Lummus, J. L., "New Material Proves Successful to Stop Lost Circulation under Various Conditions," *Petroleo Interamericano*, December 1966, p. 26.

[6]Lummus, J. L., "A New Look at Lost Circulation," *Petroleum Engineer*, November 1967, pp. 69–70, 72–3.

[7]*World Oil*, "1980–1981 Guide to Drilling, Workover, and Completion Fluids."

[8]Green, B. Q., "Eight Steps to Stop Lost Circulation," *Petroleum Engineer*, March 1963, p. 74.

[9]Billingston, S. A., "Practical Approach to Lost Circulation Problems," *Drilling Contractor*, July-August 1963, p. 52.

[10]Lummus, J. L., "Squeeze Slurries for Lost-Circulation Control," *Petroleum Engineer*, September 1968, pp. 59–64.

[11]Sheffield, J. Riley, Jr., "New $CaCO_2$ Lost Return Sealing Slurry Looks Good," *World Oil*, October 1965, pp. 133–139.

[12]Cagle, W. S., and H. Dan Mathews, "An Improved Lost Circulation Slurry Squeeze," *Petroleum Engineer*, July 1977, pp. 26, 28–9.

[13]Lummus, J. L., op cit.

[14]Clancy, Lucian W., and Manual Boudreaux, Jr., "High-Water-Loss High-Solids Slurry Stops Lost Circulation with Oil Muds," *Oil & Gas Journal*, January 5, 1981, pp. 99–101.

[15]Messenger, Joseph U., "Technique for Controlling Lost Circulation Employing Improved Soft Plug," U.S. Patent 4,183,199, issued November 13, 1979.

[16]———, "Method of Alleviating Lost Circulation," U.S. Patent 3,876,006, issued April 8, 1975.

[17]Dawson, D. D., and W. C. Goins Jr., "Bentonite-Diesel Oil Squeeze," *World Oil*, October 1953, p. 222.

[18]W. C. Goins et al., "Method of and Composition for Sealing Lost Circulation in Wells, U.S. Patent 2,900,016, issued June 27, 1961.

[19]Goins W. C. Jr., "How to Combat Circulation Loss," *Oil & Gas Journal*, June 9, 1952, pp. 71–92.

[20]*Oil & Gas Journal*, "New Gum Slurry Works Fast to Control Lost Circulation," April 25, 1966, p. 172.

[21]Vial, C. O., and V. Smith, "New Developments in Air-Gas Drilling and Completions," *World Oil*, December 1963, p. 82.

[22]Ragland, D., and G. E. Cannon, "Method of Drilling Wells," U.S. Patent 2,726,063, issued December 6, 1955.

[23]Murray, J. W., "Parasite Tubing String Solves Lost-Circulation Problems," *Oil & Gas Journal*, May 27, 1968, pp. 87–90.

SUGGESTIONS FOR FURTHER READING

Boatman, W. A., Jr. "Drill Cuttings Give Pressure Clues." *Oil & Gas Journal.* May 29, 1967, p. 66.

Everett, R. H., and L. R. Records. "Well-Killing Tool Scores Big." *Oil & Gas Journal.* June 29, 1964, p. 52.

Hottman, C. E., and J. R. Johnson. "Estimation of Formation Pressures from Log-Derived Shale Properties." *Journal of Petroleum Technology.* June 1965, p. 717.

Jorden, J. T., and O. J. Shirley. "Application of Drilling Performance Data to Overpressure Detection." *Journal of Petroleum Technology.* November 1966, p. 1387.

Kelly, John, Jr. "Lost Circulation Control." U.S. Patent 3,467,208, issued September 16,1969.

———. "Method of Controlling Lost Circulation." U.S. Patent 3,724,565, issued April 1973.

Mathews, W. R., and John Kelly Jr. "How to Predict Formation Pressure and Fracture Gradient." *Oil & Gas Journal.* February 20, 1967, p. 92.

Messenger, Joseph U. "Barite Plugs Simplify Well Control." *World Oil.* June 1969, pp. 83–85.

———. "Barite Plugs can Effectively Seal Active Zones." *Oil & Gas Journal.* April 28, 1969, pp. 67–70.

———. "Formation of Plugs within Wells." U.S. Patent 3,490,535, issued January 20, 1970.

———. "Lost Circulation Control." U.S. Patent 3,987,855, issued October 26, 1976.

———. "Technique for Controlling Lost Circulation." Patent 3,724,564, issued April 3, 1973.

———. "Well Cementing Process Using Presheared Water Swellable Clays." U.S. Patent 4,202,413, issued May 13, 1980.

Reynolds, E. B., "Predicting Overpressured Zone with Seismic Data." *World Oil.* October 1970, pp. 78–82.

Wallace, W. E. "Application of Electric-Log Measured Pressures to Drilling Problems and a New Simplified Chart for Well-Site Pressure Computation." *Log Analyst.* November-December 1965, p. 4.

Williams, David G. "For High-Pressure Wells: Six Tools Help You in the Selection of Protective-Casing Seats." *Oil & Gas Journal.* October 10, 1966, pp. 149–160.

INDEX

P
Pal-Mix 110-R, 33, **71**
plug
   barite, 35, 87, 88
   barite-in-oil, 35, 91, 92
   polymer, 33, **78**
   pronto, 37
   soft, 15, 17, 18, 19, 21, 33
   soft/hard, 15, **56**
plugged bit, 37
plugging agents, temporary, 97
productive zones, 97
protective casing, 11

S
SAPP, 89
seismic data, 13
shale densities, 13

sour gas, 99
squeeze pressure, 19, 39
squeeze procedure, 67
stabilized hole, 9, 98

T
temperature survey, 23
thixotropic cement, **47**
transition zones, 11, 12

U
underground blowout, 5, 7

W
warning system, driller, 9
water flow, 95, 96